Huntington's Disease

The Johns Hopkins Series in
Contemporary Medicine and Public Health

also of interest in this series:

The Management of Acute Stroke
C. M. C. Allen, M.D., M. J. G. Harrison, D.M., and D. T. Wade, M.D.

Migraine: Clinical and Research Aspects
J. N. Blau, M.D., ed.

Family Management of Schizophrenia: A Study of Clinical, Social, Family, and Economic Benefits
Ian R. H. Falloon, M.D., and others

Neuropeptides in Psychiatric and Neurological Disorders
Charles B. Nemeroff, M.D., PH.D., ed.

Sensory Deception: A Scientific Analysis of Hallucinations
Peter D. Slade and Richard Bentall

The Genetics of Mood Disorders
Ming T. Tsuang, M.D., PH.D., D.SC. and Stephen V. Faraone, PH.D.

Huntington's Disease

A DISORDER OF FAMILIES

Susan E. Folstein, M.D.

Associate Professor of Psychiatry
The Johns Hopkins University School of Medicine

The Johns Hopkins University Press

Baltimore and London

The Johns Hopkins University Press
701 West 40th Street
Baltimore, Maryland 21211
The Johns Hopkins Press Ltd., London

The paper used in this publication meets
the minimum requirements of American
National Standard for Information Sciences
—Permanence of Paper for Printed Library
Materials, ANSI Z39.48–1984.

Library of Congress Cataloging-in-Publication Data

Folstein, Susan E., 1944–
  Huntington's Disease.

  (The Johns Hopkins series in contemporary medicine and public
health)
  Bibliography: p.
  Includes index.
  1. Huntington's chorea. I. Title. II. Series.
[DNLM: 1. Huntington Chorea. WL 390 F671h] and public health)
RC394.H85F64 1989   616.8′51   89-11111
ISBN 0-8018-3860-6 (alk. paper)

To the many Huntington's disease patients
and their families who have helped with our research
at the Baltimore Huntington's Disease Project

Contents

Preface

This book evolved from my work, beginning in 1980, as the clinical director of the Baltimore Huntington's Disease Project (BHDP), the Huntington's disease (HD) center at the Johns Hopkins University. The staff and I developed the BHDP Research Clinic, at which clinicians currently see more than 400 HD patients each year, many of whom we have followed since 1976. The BHDP carried out a survey of HD in Maryland from 1980 to 1983 (Folstein et al. 1986, 1987). During the survey we examined patients at home and in institutions to document the clinical features of the spectrum of HD from its earliest manifestations to its most advanced state. The BHDP Research Clinic began as an efficient, systematic vehicle for evaluating cases ascertained during the survey. In our effort to gain an appreciation of the course of the illness in affected individuals, we continue to follow patients ascertained by the survey until death and autopsy.

An important purpose of the BHDP Research Clinic is to maintain current clinical documentation for a large number of patients and families who wish to participate in the research projects supported by the BHDP and by investigators in other institutions. In the course of facilitating the participation of patients in research, I have become involved in many HD research projects in psychology, neurology, genetics, pathology, and neuroscience, as well as in psychiatry, which is my primary interest. This collaborative work has provided me with experience in several types of HD research and their methods.

The primary intent of this book is to communicate current knowledge about HD—including clinical care, clinical research, and basic research—to clinicians, who may be called upon to evaluate or care for patients with HD and their families, and to researchers beginning work on HD. Because clinicians and scientists interested in HD come from a wide variety of backgrounds, it has been difficult to make each aspect of HD understandable to every likely reader and at the same time avoid boring those who may be expert in some aspects of HD research or clinical care. Compromises have been necessary, and not all readers will find all the chapters equally useful. For example, geneticists are likely to be well aware of the material in chapter 7 on genetics, but should find considerable information in other chapters that will help to broaden their knowledge of this multifaceted disorder. Although members of Huntington's disease families will find some chapters to be too technical, other chapters will provide them with useful information about diagnosis, care, and treatment.

The book begins with an introductory chapter, which outlines the history of HD, briefly describes the clinical features, and summarizes the development of HD research during this century. The remaining nine chapters are divided into three sections. The first section includes three chapters on the clinical characteristics of HD: the motor disorder, the dementia, and the emotional features. The clinical features are documented in most cases by empirical study but occasionally only by the clinical experience of the author and others. The second section is comprised of three chapters on clinical and basic research findings in the areas of neuropathology and neuroscience, epidemiology, and genetics. These chapters draw on the work of many distinguished investigators who have made important discoveries about HD in the past decade, the excitement of which I hope to have captured in terminology understandable to the clinician. The third section includes three chapters on issues of diagnosis and care: the diagnosis of HD, available treatments and a summary of experimental therapeutic trials, and counseling and presymptomatic testing for persons at risk for HD.

Each chapter, except the first, includes a case example based on a BHDP patient or family. Names and some personal details have been altered to protect confidentiality. Pedigrees used to exemplify certain aspects of HD have likewise been altered. Specifically, persons affected but undiagnosed have either been omitted or presented as unaffected.

I do not take responsibility for recommending dosages of medications: physicians should use their experience and judgment in prescribing, particularly for new and rarely used drugs.

Many people have helped in the preparation of this book. I am particularly grateful to Dr. J. Robert Cockrell, Dr. Phillip R. Slavney, Margaret H. Abbott, and Marie Killilea for their editorial suggestions and to Drs. Mahlon DeLong and John Hedreen for their help with chapter 5 on neuroanatomy and neuropathology. Some of the ideas for patient care are those of the BHDP social worker, Mary Louise Franz. Anne McDonnell Sill was my right hand day by day in analyzing data, obtaining and checking references, preparing figures and tables, and keeping me organized. Drs. Paul McHugh and Marshal Folstein have been my teachers about Huntington's disease since I was a medical student, and they have influenced my conceptualization of many aspects of HD. Finally, I thank all the HD families who have been my teachers. Their dignity and courage in the face of untold suffering provide all the motivation researchers need to continue to look for a cure for Huntington's disease.

The preparation of this book was supported by NINCDS Grant NS 16375, and by the Foundation for the Care and Cure of Huntington's Disease.

Huntington's Disease

1

Historical Perspective and Overview

The hereditary chorea, as I shall call it, is confined to certain and fortunately few families, and has been transmitted to them, an heirloom from generations away back in the dim past. It is spoken of by those in whose veins the seeds of the disease are known to exist, with a kind of horror, and not at all alluded to except through dire necessity when it is mentioned as "that disorder."
—HUNTINGTON, 1872

George Huntington described hereditary chorea at a meeting of the Meigs and Mason Academy of Medicine at Middleport, Ohio, in 1872. His account has been quoted and reprinted many times. Although it was not the first description of the hereditary chorea that bears his name (DeJong 1973), it was the clearest and most complete. William Osler (1908) wrote of Huntington's brief paper, "In the history of medicine there are few instances in which a disease has been more accurately, more graphically or more briefly described." Huntington's own brief paper still provides the best possible introduction to Huntington's disease.

It is attended generally by all the symptoms of common chorea [Sydenham's chorea], only in an aggravated degree, hardly ever manifesting itself until adult or middle life, and then coming on gradually but surely, increasing by degrees, and often occupying years in its development, until the hapless sufferer is but a quivering wreck of his former self.

There are three marked peculiarities in this disease: 1, its hereditary nature; 2, a tendency to insanity and suicide; 3, its manifesting itself as a grave disease only in adult life.

(1) Of its hereditary nature. When either or both of the parents have shown manifestations of the disease, . . . one or more of the offspring almost invariably suffer from the disease, if they live to adult age. But if by any chance these children go through life without it, the thread is broken and the grandchildren and great-grandchildren of the original shakers may rest assured that they are free from the disease. . . . Unstable and whimsical as the disease may be in other

respects, in this it is firm, it never skips a generation to again manifest itself in another; once having yielded its claims, it never regains them. In all the families, or nearly all in which the choreic taint exists, the nervous temperament preponderates, and in my grandfather's and father's experience, which conjointly cover a period of 78 years, nervous excitement in a marked degree almost invariably attends upon every disease these people may suffer from, although they may not when in health be over nervous.

(2) The tendency to insanity, and sometimes that form of insanity which leads to suicide, is marked. I know of several instances of suicide of people suffering from this form of chorea, or who belonged to families in which the disease existed. As the disease progresses the mind becomes more or less impaired, in many amounting to insanity, while in others mind and body both gradually fail until death relieves them of their sufferings. At present I know of two married men, whose wives are living, and who are constantly making love to some young lady, not seeming to be aware that there is any impropriety in it. They are suffering from chorea to such an extent that they can hardly walk, and would be thought by a stranger to be intoxicated. They are men of about 50 years of age, but never let an opportunity to flirt with a girl go past unimproved. The effect is ridiculous in the extreme.

(3) Its third peculiarity is its coming on, at least as a grave disease, only in adult life. I do not know of a single case that has shown any marked signs of chorea before the age of thirty or forty years, while those who pass the fortieth year without symptoms of the disease, are seldom attacked. It begins as an ordinary chorea might begin, by the irregular and spasmodic action of certain muscles, as of the face, arms, etc. These movements gradually increase, when muscles hitherto unaffected take on the spasmodic action, until every muscle in the body becomes affected (except the involuntary ones), and the poor patient presents a spectacle which is anything but pleasing to witness. I have never known a recovery or even an amelioration of symptoms in this form of chorea; when once it begins it clings to the bitter end. No treatment seems to be of any avail, and indeed nowadays its end is so well known to the sufferer and his friends, that medical advice is seldom sought. It seems at least to be one of the incurables.

An Overview of the Clinical Features

From George Huntington's description, it is clear that Huntington's disease is not simply a hereditary chorea but includes a triad of clinical features: dyskinesia (including chorea and other motor abnormalities), a nonaphasic dementia, and disorders of mood and perception, particularly depression. For this reason, the use of the term *Huntington's chorea* has fallen into disuse in favor of *Huntington's disease* (HD).

Although the term had not yet been invented, Huntington clearly described an autosomal dominant mechanism of genetic transmission. This means that

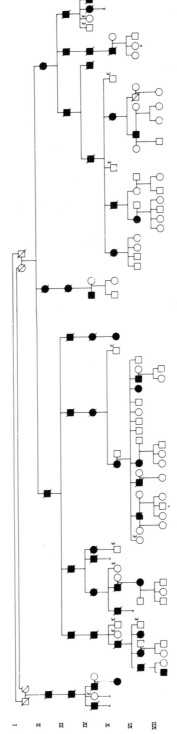

LEGEND

Males Females

□ ○	Unaffected
■ ●	Affected
■ᴇ ○ᴇ	Escaped Risk for HD: Unaffected, Living Over Age 65
⊠ ⊘	Deceased

Figure 1.1. Several branches of this large Maryland kindred were ascertained independently through affected family members. By a detailed genealogic investigation, investigators showed the numerous branches of the family to be descended from common ancestors. The family relationships were established using family reports, death certificates, wills, deeds, U.S. Census data, common surnames from state mental hospital records, and a collection of newspaper obituaries maintained by a local genealogist. Unaffected ancestors have been omitted from the figure.

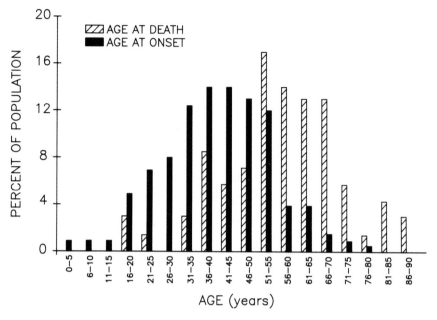

Figure 1.2. The age at the onset of Huntington's disease can vary from childhood to old age. In the Maryland survey, we defined the age at onset as the age when the family first noted motor abnormalities. The onset varied from 3 to 77 years, with the mean being 40.3 years. The age at death of the 66 patients in the survey who have died to date varied from 17 to 87 years, with a mean age of death at 56.4 years.

both males and females are equally liable, that the disease is passed from one generation to the next without skipping a generation, and that each offspring of an affected individual has a 50% chance of inheriting the HD gene and thereby the disease. If an offspring of an affected parent has not inherited the gene, he and his descendants will not have the disease. Almost all HD patients have other affected family members (implying a very low mutation rate), so with sufficient genealogic investigation, large kindreds can be documented (figure 1.1).

One inaccuracy in Huntington's description was his statement that the disease comes on only in adult life and rarely begins after the fortieth year. While this is true for the majority of patients, symptoms may begin at any time during life, from early childhood until old age (figure 1.2). The average age at onset is variously estimated to occur at 36 to 45 years of age, as Huntington observed (table 1.1). Symptoms worsen gradually, and death occurs an average of 16 years after onset, but the duration of the illness also varies widely (figure 1.3). Some patients succumb early in the illness from falls or suicide, while a few have a slowly progressive course and survive up to 40 years after choreic

Table 1.1. Mean Age at the Onset of Huntington's Disease

Study	Age of Onset	Study	Age of Onset
Bell 1934	35.5	Heathfield and	45.0
Bickford and Ellison 1953	42.8	McKenzie 1971	
		Wallace 1972	38.9
Brothers and Meadows 1955	38.3[a]	Marx 1973	35.0
		Mattsson 1974b	37.1
Reed et al. 1958	35.3[b]	Shokeir 1975a	40.5
Heathfield 1967	44.2[c]	Folstein et al.	40.3[c]
Bolt 1970	42.7[b]	1987	
Oliver 1970	36.4[b]		

[a]Changed to 35.0 in subsequent publication.
[b]Dated by chorea or behavioral change.
[c]Dated by chorea or motor impairment.

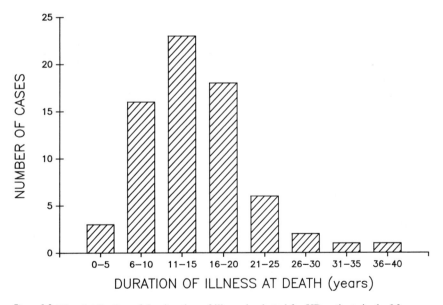

Figure 1.3. The distribution of the duration of illness is plotted for HD patients in the Maryland survey who have died. Duration of motor disorder ranged from 4 to 38 years, with the mean being 14.85 years. The estimate may be biased, because not all patients in the sample have died. The estimate based on 227 cases in the National HD Roster is 17 years (Conneally 1984).

Table 1.2. Causes of Death in 73 Huntington's Disease Patients Ascertained in a Statewide Survey

Cause of Death	N	%	Mean (SD) Duration of Illness at Death
Aspiration pneumonia	30	41	16.3 (7.3)
Cardiorespiratory failure	15	21	15.8 (7.4)
Subdural hematoma	8	11	9.8 (6.0)
Suffocation (acute)	6	8	10.2 (4.9)
Septicemia	3	4	14.3 (3.2)
Burns	2	3	6.0
Accidental strangulation	1	1	11.0
Suicide	1	1	15.0
Other (unrelated to HD)	7	10	15.4 (2.8)
Unknown	6	8	

movements begin. The most common cause of death is related to the aspiration of food into the pulmonary system, either by suffocation or by aspiration pneumonia. Causes of death in the BHDP Research Clinic series are listed in table 1.2.

While the clinical features and hereditary transmission of HD were clear from early descriptions, the neuropathologic features were not initially obvious. Early reports described a general brain softening or chronic meningitis. Jelgersma (1908) was the first to point out the major loss of neurons in the neostriatum (comprised of the caudate and putamen). In fact, although neostriatal atrophy is clearly the neuropathologic hallmark of HD, neuropathologic changes in advanced cases are widespread, as pointed out by many early writers and reviewed by Stone and Falstein in 1938.

The Origins of Huntington's Disease

Opinions vary as to why hereditary chorea was unrecognized until the mid-nineteenth century. Cases are documented in the early seventeenth century (Critchley 1973) and possibly a little earlier, but there are no convincing descriptions from ancient medicine. Perhaps the first mutation for HD occurred during the Middle Ages; perhaps the average human life span was too short for physicians to appreciate its hereditary nature; perhaps the concept of hereditary disease was too poorly developed to allow its recognition. Huntington belonged to a family of three generations of physicians practicing in the same community, providing them an unusually long time span for collective observations. One important reason that Huntington's description was quickly appreciated is that it came at a time when physicians were beginning to appreciate the concept of heredity. Mendel's laws were rediscovered shortly afterward, in 1900, and physicians were beginning to define disorders partly in terms of their hereditary features. Huntington's chorea, because its pattern of transmission was so clear, provided a model human condition that clearly followed Mendel's laws (Diefendorf's 1907 translation of Kraepelin; Osler 1908).

The populations around the world that have the highest prevalence of HD are those with roots in western Europe (Bruyn 1968; Critchley 1973; DeJong 1973). This observation, together with the low mutation rate, suggests a founder effect (Mayr 1963). When a gene is introduced by a founder (either by new mutation or by immigration) to a particular population, and when that gene has even a very slight reproductive advantage, the frequency of the gene in that population will tend to increase. Many investigators have presumed that the HD mutation occurred somewhere in northwestern Europe, was propagated there, and was later transported to other parts of the world by other founders, European explorers, and settlers. A very large proportion of recently reported Norwegian cases (Saugstad and Odegard 1986) appear to have originated in towns along the Otter River. Bruyn (1968) referred to an article by Lund, published in 1860, which described the cases in this area, and Hanssen (1914) traced one of these families back to 1550. The possibility therefore exists that the postulated founder of HD came from somewhere in Scandinavia. This is not to say that the HD mutation occurred only once or that other ethnic groups do not have HD, but the vast majority of cases throughout the world occur in populations that either originated from European migration or lived on European trade routes.

Early Research on Huntington's Disease

Shortly after 1900, papers on HD gradually began to appear in the medical literature. These included case reports and reports of clinical and pathologic features of case series. Many of these appeared in the psychiatric literature, since HD patients were cared for in psychiatric hospitals until recent years. An early survey of HD families along the eastern seaboard of the United States was undertaken by C. E. Davenport, working at the Station for Experimental Evolution in Washington, and E. V. Muncey, a member of the Eugenics Record Office at Cold Spring Harbor. The survey reported a high frequency of manic-depressive insanity in HD families, as Huntington had already pointed out (Davenport and Muncey 1916). This and many other early articles about HD took a frankly eugenic stance and suggested ways of preventing reproduction in HD families.

In 1934, Julia Bell published the first estimate of the distribution of the age at onset, based on a collection of 460 published case reports. In the late 1950s, the first systematic epidemiologic survey was undertaken by the genetics department at the University of Michigan (Reed et al. 1958; Reed and Neel 1959; Chandler, Reed, and DeJong 1960). This landmark study established the prevalence at about 4 to 5 per 100,000 population and examined a number of genetic and social issues. In 1966, Myrianthopoulos reviewed the current knowledge about HD and posed a number of important unanswered questions reflecting the paucity of information then available about HD. In 1968, Bruyn published the first comprehensive review of all the HD literature up to that time in the *Handbook of Clinical Neurology*.

The State of Knowledge 100 Years after George Huntington's Paper

The first symposium devoted to HD was held as part of a larger conference on neurogenetics in 1967. Twenty papers were given (Barbeau and Brunette 1969), including the first report pointing out that when HD began during childhood it was usually inherited from the father (Merritt et al. 1969). This was a time of great optimism for HD research because of the recent discovery that L-DOPA could reverse the symptoms of Parkinson's disease (PD). At that time, HD was considered a "mirror image" of PD, and clinicians and neuroscientists were hopeful that, using the L-DOPA replacement paradigm, they would find a treatment for HD. Even more important than the papers presented was the formation at that symposium of two complementary groups. Andre Barbeau organized the HD Research Group of the World Federation of Neurology. At the same time, the first lay organizations were established: the Committee to Combat Huntington's Disease (CCHD) was organized by Marjorie Guthrie, widow of folksinger Woodie Guthrie who had died of HD in 1967 (Klein 1980); and the Huntington's Chorea Foundation (HCF), later called the Wills Foundation, was organized to support HD research.

The HD Research Group began to meet regularly. It gradually developed research ideas, and members began to apply for research grants. At the same time, Marjorie Guthrie was organizing CCHD chapters across the country and lobbying for the recognition of HD as an important neurogenetic problem deserving research funding.

By 1972, the 100th anniversary of George Huntington's presentation of his paper *On Chorea* to the Meigs and Mason Academy of Medicine at Middleport, Ohio, enough researchers and clinicians had become interested in HD to organize a meeting devoted entirely to HD, with 146 contributors. The meeting was funded, in part, by the lay organizations (CCHD and HCF) and by the National Institute of Neurological and Communicative Diseases and Stroke (NINCDS), reflecting the early success at fundraising that was important in providing impetus for HD research.

Eighty-seven papers presented at the Centenary Symposium were collected in the first volume of *Advances in Neurology* (Barbeau, Chase, and Paulson 1973). The papers covered a range of topics that continue to occupy HD researchers today: diagnosis, clinical differences between families, nature and meaning of the emotional and cognitive abnormalities, effect of HD on the family and the community, paternal transmission effect, estimation of preva-

lence, methods for presymptomatic detection, clinical-pathologic relationships, pathophysiology, and the need for an animal model of HD. The depletion
of γ-aminobutyric acid (GABA) in the striatum was first described (Perry et al.
1973) at this symposium, and two early attempts at using genetic linkage to find
the HD gene were reported (Lindstrom et al. 1973; Beckman et al. 1973).

The Voluntary Organizations and the Congressional Commission

The pace of HD-related research accelerated after 1972, as reflected in the
increase in *Index Medicus* citations from an average of 36 per year in 1970 to
more than 100 per year in 1978. This number has remained steady to the
present, with shifts in topics as new discoveries have been made. Simultane-
ously, the voluntary organizations continued to educate the public, raise funds,
and, in the United States, exert political pressure on Congress. An important
outcome was the creation by Congress in 1975 of the Commission for the
Control of Huntington's Disease and Its Consequences. Marjorie Guthrie
served as chairperson of the commission, and the executive director was Dr.
Nancy Wexler, a clinical psychologist whose mother was afflicted with HD.
(Her father, Dr. Milton Wexler, established the Hereditary Disease Foundation
to promote research in HD.) As executive director of the commission, Dr.
Wexler brought together many scientists and clinicians who had some knowledge of HD and organized them into working groups, each assigned to a
particular topic relevant to research or treatment. At the same time, she held
gatherings around the United States to collect testimony from affected families
as a means of documenting for Congress the magnitude of the burden of HD.
The result was a report (U.S. DHEW 1977) presented to Congress along with a
film illustrating the symptoms and course of HD. The report included the
testimony of families, a collection of reports from the working groups describing the state of knowledge about HD, and recommendations for action.

The Implementation of the Recommendations of the Congressional Commission

Perhaps unique in the history of congressional commissions, and clearly a
testimony to the energy and determination of Dr. Nancy Wexler, all of the
major recommendations were eventually implemented. The recommendations
included a convocation of scientists involved in HD research, which took place
in San Diego in November 1978 (Chase, Wexler, and Barbeau 1979). At this
time HD research focused on improved diagnostic methods and clearer defini-
tions of motor, cognitive, and psychiatric features, genetic linkage studies,
striatal physiology, and endocrinologic, immunologic, and cell membrane pathology. More advances had been made in defining the abnormalities of neu-
roreceptors and transmitters, an animal model had been developed using excitotoxins, and numerous (although unsuccessful) drug treatment trials were

reported. The 1978 conference clearly demonstrated that a critical mass of expert investigators was devoting a high level of energy and talent to unraveling the mysteries of HD.

In the United States this research effort has grown even larger today as a result of the implementation of the other recommendations of the congressional commission. A National Roster for HD was established in 1979, under the direction of Dr. Michael Conneally at the University of Indiana, facilitating research requiring large or specialized samples of HD patients. In 1980 the NINCDS funded two national centers for HD research: one at Harvard in collaboration with Boston University and MIT, and the other at Johns Hopkins in Baltimore. Both have made advances in epidemiology, psychiatry, psychology, genetics, neuroscience, and patient care in HD.

Another of the commission's recommendations was the study of a large Venezuelan HD family. Under the leadership of Dr. Wexler, a team of clinicians documented the genealogy, examined all the family members, and obtained blood samples. DNA extracted from these samples was used by Dr. James Gusella in the genetic linkage study that resulted in the discovery of the locus of the HD gene and the availability of presymptomatic testing for HD (Gusella et al. 1983).

In addition to research funded as a direct result of the commission, several other medical institutions in the United States have major research and clinical commitments to HD, including the intramural branch of the NIH, the Universities of Rochester, Michigan, Chicago, and Oregon, Columbia University, and Emory University. Two brain banks, at the Los Angeles Veterans Administration Medical Center (Dr. W. W. Tourtellotte) and McLean Hospital at Harvard (Dr. E. W. Bird), have large collections of brains from HD patients and make them available to investigators. Equally important HD research groups are currently active in Canada at the University of British Columbia and in Great Britain at the National University of Wales, Cambridge University, and Leeds University. European universities with active HD research groups include the Universities of Leyden, Louvain, Vienna, and Dusseldorf. In Australia, groups are active in New South Wales and in Victoria. In addition, individual investigators continue to make important contributions relevant to HD, particularly in basic neuroscience and genetics.

I

THE TRIAD OF CLINICAL FEATURES

2

The Motor Disorder

The hereditary chorea . . . is attended generally by all the symptoms of common chorea, only in an aggravated degree.
—HUNTINGTON, 1872

The disorder of movement in Huntington's disease has two components: involuntary movements and abnormalities of voluntary movement. The involuntary movements are most commonly choreic, but motor restlessness, myoclonus, dystonia, and athetosis may also be seen. Voluntary movement is impaired by clumsiness, bradykinesia, slowing of response time, and the inability to sustain a voluntary movement, and is thus similar in some ways to parkinsonism. Involuntary movements usually predominate early in the illness, but these may gradually diminish late in the course, giving way to a rigid akinetic state.

This chapter describes the motor disorder in HD as it presents in the community and in the clinic, details the varieties of voluntary and involuntary movement that can occur, discusses the evidence from physiologic and pharmacologic studies that these constitute two separate movement disorders, and introduces current concepts of the neurophysiologic basis of abnormal movements in HD.

Case Example: The Development of the Movement Disorder of HD

Mrs. Dawson,* a married woman at 50% risk for HD, held a responsible position as an administrative secretary and advanced steadily in the company over the ten years of her employment. She was examined yearly at the BHDP Research Clinic as a research volunteer. Her first two annual neurologic examinations were normal, although at her second visit she complained of intermittent dysphoria, which she attributed to marital stress.

At her third visit, age 32, Mrs. Dawson reported that she had been in psychotherapy because of persistent emotional distress and domestic difficulties. She denied having problems at work, but said she needed to keep detailed

*Mrs. Dawson is a composite of two patients.

notes to remember all her assignments for the day. On examination, she showed mild dystonic posturing of one hand during conversation and mild motor restlessness. With her eyes closed and arms extended at 90°, she had intermittent, low-amplitude movements of her fingers.

A few months later, Mrs. Dawson reported that her employer had threatened to fire her if the quality and quantity of her work did not improve; she wondered if she might be getting HD. When examined during this period of extreme stress, she had, in addition to the previous findings, slight facial twitching and mildly dysrhythmic finger-thumb tapping. During heel-to-toe walking, she made two side steps to regain her balance. CT scan was normal (as would be expected so early in the course of illness), and thyroid function tests showed normal values (thereby ruling out thyroid disease as a cause of her involuntary movements). A diagnosis of HD was made.

By age 35, three years after onset, Mrs. Dawson's choreic movements were more widespread and were rated 2/5 (with 5 as the most severe rating; see Appendix 1 for ratings) during most activities, increasing to 3/5 (some high-amplitude jerks) when she was stressed, either by an emotionally laden topic or by performing mental arithmetic. Her speech was mildly dysrhythmic and became more hesitant when she discussed complicated topics. Saccades, or quick, voluntary eye movements, were mildly slow, and she required intense concentration to suppress blinking and head movements while moving her eyes quickly from side to side. She could mimic most facial movements, such as puffing out her cheeks, winking, and frowning, but she could not move her tongue rapidly from side to side. Muscle tone was slightly decreased, and deep tendon reflexes were brisk, though without clonus. Finger-thumb tapping and rapid alternating movements of the hands were arrhythmic and a little slow. She held her hands in an awkward dystonic posture while performing these tasks. Finger-to-nose movements were slightly awkward but not dysmetric. She could stand with her feet together, but her gait was slightly widely based, and she accomplished ten tandem steps, heel-to-toe, with difficulty.

At home Mrs. Dawson still cared for the house, although the work went more slowly. Meal planning and execution were becoming slightly disorganized, and she had several horizontal scars on the inner aspects of her forearms where she had burned herself while taking food from the oven. At this time she was advised to request help when using the oven and to stop driving a car.

Seven years after onset, the early neurologic findings were more severe, and new signs had appeared. Her speech, while understandable, was markedly dysrhythmic and slow, and associated with chorea and dystonic posturing of her arms and trunk. Topics of conversation were simple ones. Her chorea was now rated 3/5 during conversation and while performing a motor task. She could voluntarily inhibit this chorea to 2/5 upon request, but when she was stressed the movements became constant and of very high amplitude with a 4/5 rating. She had marked difficulty mimicking facial movements and became dystonic in the attempt. Tone varied and was sometimes increased throughout the range of movement. Deep tendon reflexes could be elicited with the slightest tap, and unsustained ankle clonus was present. Her gait was widely based, with reeling from side to side, unexpected knee bends, and small steps. Turning was awkward and performed carefully to avoid a fall; she could not complete heel-to-toe walking for fear of a fall.

Mrs. Dawson now required minor assistance with grooming and dressing and had to purchase clothes without buttons or zippers. Household duties had been assumed by other family members. This change was instituted after Mrs. Dawson fell down the steps while carrying laundry and later caused a kitchen fire because she forgot she had bacon frying. She could no longer concentrate on complex reading, but kept up with current events through television.

Ten years after onset, the constellation of neurologic signs had changed slightly. Although the chorea was rated only marginally worse than at year seven, the voluntary motor abnormalities had worsened considerably. Speech was quite slow and difficult to understand, and the effort of speaking worsened the involuntary movements, both choreic and dystonic. Voluntary eye movements were possible only with a preceding head thrust and were very slow. The eyes moved slightly better in pursuit of a target, but the movement was broken down into several small movements, and it was difficult for Mrs. Dawson to maintain her attention on the target. She was unable to keep her eyes closed upon command or voluntarily protrude her tongue. She could not even attempt to mimic facial movements. Tone was increased throughout the range of motion, reflexes were brisk with clonus, and the right plantar response was extensor. Strength was mildly decreased. She perceived how to perform finger-thumb tapping and rapid alternating movements, but had great difficulty moving her hands to perform them. She could walk independently at home and in the clinic for short distances, but her husband insisted that she use a wheelchair when leaving the house. Her gait was stiff-legged and very widely based, and she extended her arms laterally to avoid falling backward. This was her last visit to the clinic, because it had become too difficult for her to leave the house.

When examined at a home visit 13 years after onset, Mrs. Dawson could barely speak, although she recognized the clinic nurse and retained her interest in particular television programs. She was fed a soft diet, and all her daily needs were met by others. Regular toileting prevented incontinence. She spent most of her time in a padded hospital bed, finding long periods in a chair too exhausting. She expressed displeasure by screaming.

When undisturbed by visitors, she had no involuntary movement. Any stimulation, regardless of its nature, precipitated stiff-limbed, flailing movements. She was alert and appeared to take an interest in the examination. She lay in bed with her legs and ankles extended. One arm and hand were flexed and the other extended. Her eyes remained midposition, and she sometimes moved her head to follow the examiner's movements about the room. She could not perform any voluntary movements upon request, although sometimes she appeared to be making an attempt. Tone was markedly increased, making it almost impossible to move her limbs or elicit deep tendon reflexes. Plantar responses were extensor, bilaterally.

The Presentation of the Motor Disorder at Home and at Work

For several years before seeking treatment, an affected person may be unable to maintain even pressure on the accelerator of a car, may tap a foot in church or other places where restlessness is socially embarrassing, or may have ticlike movements of an eye, a shoulder, or some other isolated muscle group. The person may not notice these mild movements and the family may not seek medical attention for them, unless they are aware of a risk for HD. Later, the person may become more restless, with increased gesticulation and excessive movements while seated. Some may experience unexpected falls, claiming that their knees suddenly give way or that they trip over curbs. Next, clumsiness with tools or household items begins, along with dropping things. By this time, the family may notice that the person is slightly slower in speech and less efficient in the performance of such daily activities as dressing, shaving, preparing meals, or making home repairs. These signs cause concern and usually result in seeking medical consultation.

As the illness becomes well developed, obvious involuntary movements occur, usually jerky, unpredictable, choreic movements that have a characteristic pattern for an individual patient. Patients may be referred to a physician by their employer for suspected alcohol intoxication at work or because of injury (or fear of injury) on the job. At the same time, voluntary actions are becoming clumsy and slow, which also interfere with job performance.

Both voluntary and involuntary movements gradually worsen over many years. Eventually they affect the ability to speak, walk, and eat. Dysarthria, initially noticed as a slowness and dysrhythmia of speech, becomes so severe that the patient's requests are difficult to understand. Balance is affected both by unexpected choreic jerks and by increasing muscle tone, so falls become a constant worry, and the patient becomes confined to a chair and then to bed. Similarly eating is compromised by both chorea (unexpected breaths while swallowing which result in aspiration) and a decreased ability to chew and swallow. The risk of choking on food gradually increases. By this time the patient requires considerable assistance with dressing and grooming and cannot be left unattended. After about 13 to 15 years of illness, the average patient requires total care.

The Presentation of the Motor Disorder in the Clinic

In a person with mild motor signs who may present with complaints of depression or trouble functioning at work, a formal examination of the motor system may show little abnormality. Mild involuntary movements may be noticed only when the patient is severely stressed, as when greeting the physician or doing mental calculations. Commonly, upon being greeted by the physician, the patient will rise from the chair with an awkward whole-body movement, looking as though he might lose his balance. His handshake may be abnormal, with a sudden squeeze and quick release (the "milkmaid's sign"). During history taking, the patient should be observed constantly for *involuntary* motor abnormalities. Except for bradykinesia, abnormalities of *voluntary* movement are more readily observed during a formal neurologic examination. The BHDP Research Clinic developed a quantified version of the clinical neurologic examination of the motor systems for use in our research clinic (Folstein, Jensen et al. 1983; David et al. 1987). The format and instructions for its use are included in Appendix 1.

Involuntary Movements

A variety of involuntary movements occur in HD. While chorea is most common, motor restlessness, dystonia, tremor, and myoclonus may also be present, and it is not clear whether these involuntary movements have the same or different pathophysiologic mechanisms. Marsden (1984) reported that HD patients with chorea can have electromyograms typical for chorea, myoclonus, or dystonia. Clinically the chorea, myoclonus, and dystonia are quite different, and it is important to recognize that all may be seen in HD, sometimes in the same patient either at the same examination or at different times during the course of illness. In some patients, chorea never predominates. The form of HD with mild or absent chorea, akinesia, and hypertonia is called the Westphal variant (reviewed by Bruyn 1968). It is most common in children and adolescents but is occasionally seen in adults. In adults, marked akinesia may or may not be accompanied by hypertonia.

Chorea   Chorea, meaning "dance," is characterized by sudden, quick, unintended movements of almost any part of the body. Unlike tics, chorea is not stereotyped and repetitive, nor limited to a particular body part. Early in the illness, choreic movements are usually low in amplitude and occur in distal body parts, especially the hands and feet. However, some patients begin with proximal involuntary movements of the trunk or shoulder. As time passes, the movements become more frequent and pervasive and of higher amplitude, usually reaching a peak of severity about 10 years after onset. Following this, involuntary movements either plateau or lessen and may disappear in patients who survive for 15 years, except when the patient is stimulated (figure 2.1; Folstein, Jensen et al. 1983, Folstein et al. 1986).

A few patients—most commonly those with onset before age 20—never have chorea. In a surprising number of adults, chorea never reaches the high amplitude and intensity usually presented as typical (table 2.1).

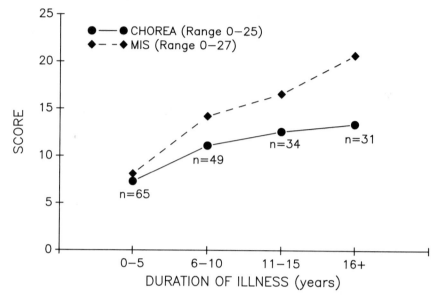

Figure 2.1. Chorea and MIS plotted by duration groups. A factor analysis of a quantified version of the clinical neurologic examination of the motor system revealed two independent scales: the chorea scale (score 0–25) and the motor impairment scale, or MIS, (score 0–27) composed mainly of items testing voluntary movements. While the MIS scores worsen predictably over time, chorea scores plateau after several years of illness (Folstein, Jensen et al. 1983).

Table 2.1. Severity of Chorea in Huntington's Disease Patients
(Distribution by Percentage within Each Duration-of-Illness Group)

Severity of Chorea	Years since the Onset of Chorea					
	0–3	4–7	8–11	12–15	16–19	20+
Absent	0	12	11	0	8	0
Mild	76	27	14	8	0	0
Moderate	18	55	49	72	61	60
Severe	6	6	26	20	31	40
	(N = 34)	(N = 32)	(N = 35)	(N = 25)	(N = 13)	(N = 10)

Note: Although chorea is usually present, nine patients had no chorea at the time of examination. Severe chorea was found in fewer than half the patients who had been ill between 12 and 20 years. Chorea was rated in five settings: at rest, during conversation, during a standard voluntary motor task, with arms outstretched at 90°, and during a stressful activity. Scores for each setting ranged from 0 to 5, and were summed to give a chorea score of 0 to 25. Scores of 1 to 8 were called mild, 9 to 16 moderate, and 17 to 25 severe.

Voluntary movement and psychological stress influence the expression of chorea differently. Chorea is worsened by a stressful task such as counting backward by seven and lessened by voluntary movements such as writing or walking (figure 2.2). It can also be decreased by intense concentration. At the onset of illness, chorea may be apparent only when the patient is stressed by describing symptoms to the physician, by being asked to calculate, or by attempting to recall the dates of life events. In very late HD, when chorea has diminished overall, it increases when the patient is stimulated or attempts to make a voluntary movement.

The chorea of HD is somewhat different from that seen in Sydenham's chorea (a late manifestation of streptococcal infection). The movements in HD are not as quick and lightninglike as those seen in Sydenham's chorea (Osler 1894). In addition, chorea in HD frequently has a writing quality, further along on the continuum toward athetosis.

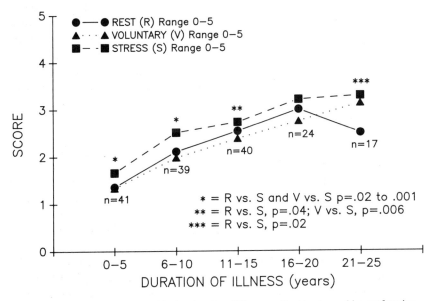

Figure 2.2. Chorea ratings vary with the situation. When a patient is stressed by performing a difficult task or discussing an emotionally laden topic (*Stress*), chorea is worse than when the patient is executing a motor task (*Voluntary*) or is asked to relax and hold perfectly still (*Rest*). These differences are significant for patients who were examined during the first half of the course of illness. In later years (16 years of illness or more) those patients *who could be scored* on all chorea measures could not voluntarily stop their movements, which were significantly less only when the patient was at rest. Patients who could not perform voluntary movements were excluded from the analysis (unpublished data).

Motor Restlessness   Before the onset of choreic movements, patients often have motor restlessness. Families comment that patients gesticulate more, are unable to sit quietly, and appear anxious or nervous. Patients themselves are largely unaware of this movement. Physicians' notes comment on such restlessness, at the same time remarking that chorea was not observed. Contrary to the common teaching, chorea and motor restlessness can also be present during sleep. Spouses notice that the bed is torn apart during sleep, and they observe excessive movement while the patient is in a deep sleep. These movements may be present for several years before the onset of clinically observable chorea. The patient is unaware of these movements and denies having restless nights.

Dystonia   Dystonic posturing can coexist with chorea or motor restlessness or may be seen alone. Early in the illness, patients may hold an arm, a leg, or the upper body in an awkward position. For example, the leg may be raised off the floor, with the foot adducted. Similarly, the forearm may be held up, with the hand flexed or extended. These postures often involve only one side of the body and are usually observed while the patient is concentrating on a voluntary motor task or conversation. Dystonia may be seen in any patient at any time during the course, but it is most severe and prominent in juvenile-onset cases with the Westphal variant and in patients with advanced disease. After several years of severe dystonia, the body becomes permanently twisted. Children with the Westphal variant often develop scoliosis. Lugaresi, Cirignotta, and Montagna (1986) reported a patient with HD who had nocturnal dystonic attacks years before the onset of other symptoms.

Tremor and Myoclonic Jerks   Persons at risk for HD may display a fine tremor when they hold their arms extended, but its significance is unclear. In our experience, it often appears to be related to caffeine, alcohol, or other drug intake, and it is not observed consistently from year to year. A coarse tremor can be seen in patients with the Westphal variant. This tremor can involve either the head or the limbs and occurs both at rest and during voluntary motor activity.

Myoclonic jerks are rare but can be seen in children and adolescents with HD and patients with advanced disease. In a few patients tapping a reflex or touching may cause sustained whole-body myoclonus. Family members sometimes report these waves of myoclonus as seizures.

In summary, chorea is by far the most common involuntary movement seen in HD, although severity varies considerably from case to case. Motor restlessness can precede frank chorea. Mild dystonia commonly accompanies chorea and motor restlessness; but dystonia may become severe (as may tremor and myoclonus) in patients with the Westphal variant and those with advanced disease.

Abnormalities of Voluntary Movement

Parkinson's disease (PD) and Huntington's disease are frequently contrasted in terms of motor speed, with PD characterized by bradykinesia and HD by hyperkinesia. This is misleading. At the same time that HD patients have hyperkinetic involuntary movements, their voluntary movements are slow.

Not only are voluntary motor acts bradykinetic and clumsy, motor activity cannot be maintained over a period of time (motor impersistence), and there is often a lag before the initiation of a voluntary movement (motor latency). Voluntary motor impairment in HD is demonstrated most clearly in the examination of eye movements and is also observed in coordination, gait, speech, and swallowing.

In contrast to chorea, which bears an unpredictable relation to the course of illness and may be absent, abnormalities of voluntary motor activity are always present and steadily worsen as the illness progresses (figure 2.1).

Eye Movements   Eye movements are of two general types (Dodge, Travis, and Fox 1930). Tracking or following movements are relatively slow (up to 45° per second) and are used to maintain gaze on a moving target. They can be considered a response to velocity. Saccades or version movements are quick (up to 60° per second), discrete movements that bring the eyes promptly to an eccentric point in the visual field and can be considered a response to position. These two types of movement have different neural mechanisms and are differentially affected in HD (Starr 1967; Leigh et al. 1983). Tracking movements are relatively preserved until midway in the illness, while impaired saccades occur very early and may precede other neurologic signs by several years (figure 2.3A). The pattern of eye movement abnormalities varies from patient to patient and findings are most dependent on the duration of the illness at the time of examination (table 2.2).

HD affects saccades in several ways. First, saccades may be slow. This abnormality is best demonstrated clinically by having the patient direct his gaze alternately between two targets at the extremes of lateral gaze. Clinical judgment is aided by asking the spouse or other clinic personnel to perform the same task. This abnormality is more easily demonstrated in the laboratory (figure 2.3C).

Second, saccades may not begin promptly (figure 2.3B). Saccadic latency is more marked when the saccade is initiated intentionally by the patient than when the movement is made reflexively in response to a sudden visual stimulus (Lasker et al. 1987). Some patients are able to initiate a saccade only if they first move their heads or blink (Leigh et al. 1983).

The third saccadic abnormality is a reduction in the distance moved, or hypometria. Some patients move the eyes laterally across the visual field in several short saccades rather than one continuous movement. Finally, it can be

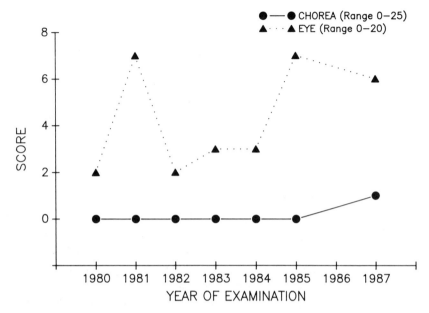

Figure 2.3. (A) Abnormal eye movements were documented at yearly clinical examinations of this at-risk person for 7 years before chorea appeared. During the 7 years, the individual was successfully employed and MMSE scores were in the normal range. By genetic testing, the individual is 99% likely to have HD.

demonstrated in the laboratory that HD patients with even minimal neurologic and cognitive symptoms cannot voluntarily suppress a saccade to a suddenly appearing visual target (Lasker et al. 1987). This experimental stressing of the eye movement system may aid in the diagnosis of HD in persons at risk who have minimal and ambiguous neurologic signs.

Tracking eye movements are usually preserved until several years after onset, but subtle impairments may be observed earlier. Some patients have trouble maintaining their gaze on a moving target (e.g., a pencil tip) and will suddenly avert their gaze. This could be interpreted as either impersistence of movement or an inability to suppress reflex saccades to a visually distracting stimulus. Inability to maintain attention on a moving target occurs less often in the laboratory, where visual pursuit is performed in the dark without visual distractions.

Eye movements are better preserved in patients whose symptoms appear later in life. Often the only clinically observable sign is latency of saccade initiation. However, in the laboratory, even patients with a normal clinical eye examination are unable to suppress reflex saccades to suddenly appearing stimuli (Lasker et al. 1988). Most patients with very advanced disease are able to

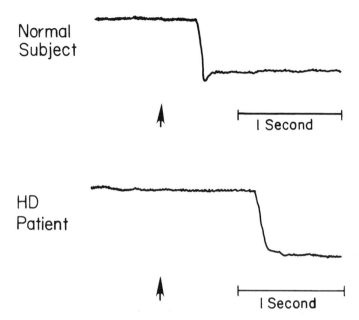

Figure 2.3. (*B*) Some HD patients have difficulty initiating saccadic eye movements, even though the movement may be of normal velocity once started. This latency of initiation is more common in patients whose illness begins late in life. The *arrow* designates the onset of the light stimulus to which the subject had been instructed to direct his gaze. In this example the age-matched normal subject made a saccade 250 milliseconds (ms) after the light came on, compared with 1000 ms for the HD patient.

move their eyes only in response to passive head movement, known as the "doll's eyes" maneuver.

Fine Motor Coordination   Patients with HD become progressively less able to use their hands for fine motor tasks (table 2.3). This appears to result from a combination of chorea and voluntary motor impairment, but it is seen in patients with only minimal chorea and is prominent in patients with the Westphal variant.

In daily life patients are clumsy, as noticed early in the illness by a loss of ability to manipulate tools or perform fine needlework. Tying shoes, buttoning clothes, and cutting food are performed awkwardly. Patients have difficulty sustaining rhythmic activities such as cutting meat and vegetables. Eventually, patients lose the use of their hands entirely.

On neurologic examination, fine motor incoordination is usually seen first in the nondominant hand (Oepen et al. 1985). This can be best appreciated in the clinic by testing finger-thumb tapping and rapid alternating hand movements. Minimally affected patients are quick but dysrhythmic on finger-thumb tap-

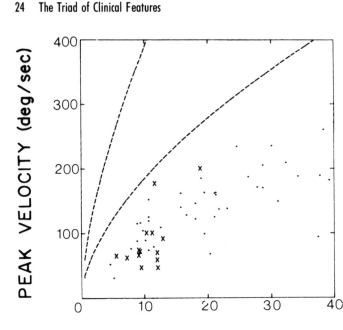

AMPLITUDE (deg)

Figure 2.3. (*C*) In normal persons, saccadic eye movements made between two points increase in velocity as the distance between the two points is increased. The normal range of velocities is demarcated by the upper and lower lines. Patients with HD are unable to increase the speed of their saccades as the distance between the targets is increased. It is easiest to demonstrate slow saccades by having the patients look alternately at two targets at the extremes of lateral gaze, instructing them to move their eyes as fast as possible. (Source: Leigh et al. 1983, reprinted with permission.)

ping. Later they become slower and cannot maintain the tapping for more than a few repetitions. In advanced disease, patients appear to perceive the task and attempt to raise an arm to initiate it, but they cannot oppose the finger and thumb. The earliest abnormality in rapid alternating hand movements is the occasional failure to maintain a steady alternation between pronation and supination. Later the dysrhythmia and slowing resemble that observed in finger-thumb tapping. Patients with little chorea (but several years into the illness) can perform rapid alternating and tapping movements more accurately than choreic patients, but their movements are slow and unsustained.

Speech   Speech is a complex activity involving thought, language, and motor behavior. In HD, aspects of these three functions are affected (Gordon and Illes 1987), and it is difficult to disentangle them. Clearly, HD patients have speech motor abnormalities of both rhythm and speed (Ramig 1986). Speech is dys-

Table 2.2. Oculomotor Abnormalities Encountered in Patients by Duration of Illness (Percentage of Patients in Group with Abnormality)

Oculomotor Abnormality	Duration of Illness (in years)			
	0–5	6–10	11–15	16+
Fixation abnormality	70	75	83	66
Impaired saccadic initiation				
Obligatory head movement	78	100	100	100
Increased latency	78	100	100	100
Obligatory blink	22	59	33	50
Slow saccades				
Vertical plane	52	67	67	83
Horizontal plane	39	50	56	83
Reduced range of saccadic movement				
Vertical plane	37	66	89	100
Horizontal plane	22	50	89	100
Smooth pursuit abnormality				
Vertical plane	52	64	67	100
Horizontal plane	48	64	57	100
Vergence abnormality	19	36	50	100
	(N = 23)	(N = 12)	(N = 9)	(N = 6)

Note: Early in the illness, the most common abnormalities of eye movements are impaired initiation and speed of saccades and impaired fixation of gaze on an eccentric point. As the illness progresses, more aspects of eye movement become abnormal, until, very late in the illness, the eyes remain fixed at midposition and move only when the examiner moves the patient's head (the "doll's eye maneuver").

rhythmic, with bursts of words and pauses in mid phrase. There is also a loss of volume at the ends of phrases. Speech is slower than normal, in terms of both the number of words produced over time and the initiation of a reply to a question. As the disease progresses, speech becomes difficult to understand and patients appear to have increasing difficulty in initiating speech. Eventually, patients stop talking altogether. The motor difficulties with speech probably result from irregular breathing and the loss of control of the tongue, combined with cognitive changes related to the speed and persistence of thought processes and the loss of ready access to memory stores. As in most nonchoreic motor abnormalities in HD, speech is not improved by medications that suppress chorea (e.g., Bassi et al. 1986).

Dysphagia   The ingestion of food involves a coordinated process of getting the food to the mouth, opening the mouth, chewing, searching the mouth with coordinated movements of the tongue and cheeks, forming a bolus, and swallowing, while at the same time inhibiting breathing. Feeding in HD is obviously

Table 2.3. Nonchoreic Motor Abnormalities in Huntington's Disease Patients (Percentage of Patients in Group with Abnormality)

Motor Abnormality	Years since the Onset of Chorea					
	0–3	4–7	8–11	12–15	16–19	20+
Rhythm and speed						
Rapid tongue movement	85	93	100	92	100	100
Finger-thumb tap (dominant hand)	79	87	100	100	100	100
Diadochokinesis (dominant hand)	79	94	94	100	100	100
Speech						
Dysrhythmia	63	90	89	92	100	100
Slow	33	65	89	96	100	100
Mild dysarthria	33	50	54	56	23	70
Severe dysarthria	0	9	20	12	23	20
Mute	0	0	9	20	54	10
Station and gait						
Abnormal posture	18	41	66	58	85	90
Cannot stand with feet together	18	48	77	80	85	80
Widely based or reeling gait	56	65	57	56	23	40
Walks with assistance or unable to walk	0	13	34	40	77	60
Abnormal tandem walking	62	72	94	92	100	100
Other motor signs						
Hypertonia	23	32	29	40	58	80
Hyperreflexia without clonus	56	40	46	36	0	20
Hyperreflexia with clonus	9	19	24	24	62	80
Extensor plantar	6	17	35	13	54	60
Bradykinesia						
Mild	65	41	50	24	8	20
Severe	9	22	38	52	77	80
	(N = 34)	(N = 32)	(N = 35)	(N = 25)	(N = 13)	(N = 10)

Note: Nonchoreic abnormalities gradually worsen with the duration of the illness. Tasks of rhythm and speed are commonly affected earliest, followed by dysarthria. Difficulty with tandem walking appears early, and most patients are unable to walk after 16 years of illness. Late signs include hypertonia and hyperreflexia and extensor influenced by chorea, coordination of the various voluntary motor acts involved, and hunger.

Feeding is characterized by spilling (proportional to the severity of chorea), filling the mouth too full before swallowing (patients say they are very hungry), and choking (because of the failure to coordinate chewing and swallowing with suppression of breathing). Chewing is arrhythmic and tongue movements are poorly coordinated and ineffective in moving the food toward the back of the mouth. Swallowing is hampered by poorly coordinated movements of the mouth and pharynx and by unexpected inspirations during swallowing, which induce coughing and aspiration (Leopold and Kagel 1985). Aspiration of food is the most common cause of death in HD. Forty-nine percent of patients ascertained in the Maryland survey died from suffocation on a food bolus or from aspiration pneumonia (table 1.2).

Gait   Patients with HD have a widely based, somewhat slow gait, take short steps, and have difficulty turning on a pivot (see table 2.3). The cadence or rhythm of their steps is irregular and they may suddenly bend the knee in an exaggerated way (Koller and Trimble 1985). Some aspects of the gait disturbance are related to chorea, particularly the sudden knee bends that are seen only in choreic patients. However, most aspects of gait appear to be unrelated to chorea. Walking speed and balance (as examined in heel-to-toe walking) can be impaired in patients with minimal chorea, and the gait is usually widely based. Patients with the Westphal variant have a more spastic, stiff-legged, widely based gait and early trouble with tandem walking. On the other hand, some patients with quite severe chorea can tandem walk without losing their balance. Many patients automatically suppress choreic movements when concentrating on walking, but this decrease in involuntary movement does not permit them to narrow their base or perform tandem walking. In addition, medications such as haloperidol which suppress chorea do not improve the gait (Koller and Trimble 1985; Nutt and Morgan 1983).

About 10 years after onset, walking becomes very difficult. In the BHDP survey sample, nearly half the patients who had been ill for 10 years were unable to walk without assistance; only 6% of patients could walk after 16 years of illness. Patients at this stage who can walk proceed slowly with short steps, a markedly wide base, and great lurches followed by attempts to regain balance. They turn with several careful shuffling steps. Falls become common and life-threatening, with the risk of death due to a subdural hematoma. When difficulty with walking becomes severe, muscle tone is usually increased, with brisk deep tendon reflexes and ankle clonus.

Motor Findings in End-Stage HD

Toward the end of life, involuntary movements usually lessen, leaving the patient in a state of akinetic mutism. Some family members describe patients in this state as "locked into their bodies." The patients have also been cited as examples of a persistent vegetative state (Walshe and Leonard 1985). Many patients recognize family members and respond briefly to their presence or to news of other relatives, but these responses are sustained only fleetingly, and then the patients lapse back into unresponsiveness or may stare ahead at a television set. Other patients do not respond at all, and a few actively resist any attempted communication or bodily contact.

Physical examination is characterized by occasional, involuntary, whole-limb movements that resemble myoclonus. The movements may occur only when the patient is agitated. Eyes move very little, except when the head is moved passively from side to side. Most patients are mute, although caretakers report rare utterances made in response to marked emotional provocation. Muscle tone is usually very rigid, and joint contractures of all extremities are commonly present. For this reason, reflexes may be hard to elicit, but if present they are very brisk with sustained ankle clonus and positive Babinski signs. Many patients also have snout and grasp reflexes. Even patients who are interested in cooperating with examination are unable to execute any voluntary movements, although their attempts often indicate an understanding of what is requested. Most patients who survive to this stage are unable to swallow and must be fed via gastrostomy or nasogastric tube.

The Experimental Evidence for the Distinction between Voluntary and Involuntary Movements

In the clinic, voluntary motor abnormalities can be difficult to detect in patients with severe chorea, and clinical accounts often describe voluntary movements as interrupted by chorea. Falls and choking also tend to be attributed to involuntary movement. However, several lines of evidence suggest that voluntary and involuntary movements are distinguishable on clinical and pathophysiologic grounds.

First, HD patients with the Westphal variant have little or no chorea. In contrast with hyperkinetic HD patients, they have increased muscle tone and paucity of movement (rigid and akinetic). However, they have the same difficulties with speech, swallowing, fine motor coordination, and gait as hyperkinetic HD patients, suggesting that these difficulties cannot be ascribed to chorea.

Second, there are different clinical correlates with voluntary and involuntary movements. When the Quantified Neurologic Examination (QNE) was subjected to factor analysis, the chorea items formed one factor (the chorea subscale), which was independent of a second factor formed by several items measuring voluntary motor impairment (the motor impairment subscale; Folstein, Jensen et al. 1983). Moreover, when these two subscales were correlated with duration of illness, cognitive capacity, and activities of daily living, the

Table 2.4. Relationship between Involuntary and Voluntary Movements and Measures of Cognition and Social Function

Test	Chorea Score	Motor Impairment Score
Mini-Mental score	0.43 (N = 177)	0.80 (N = 168)
Activities of Daily Living score	0.41 (N = 173)	0.71 (N = 164)

Note: While clinical ratings of both chorea and voluntary motor impairment (MIS) are significantly correlated with MMSE scores and with general functioning (activities of daily living), the correlations of the MIS with these functions are much higher.

correlations were different. Voluntary motor impairment correlated much more strongly with these measures of the severity of illness than did the chorea scale (table 2.4).

A third useful contrast may be made between HD and tardive dyskinesia

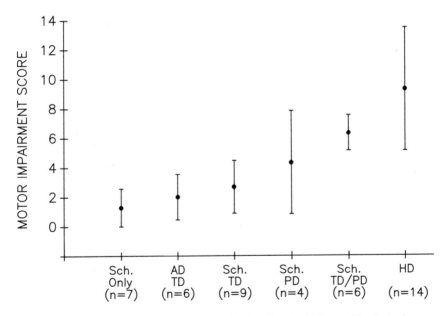

Figure 2.4. Patients with schizophrenia (*SCH*), affective disorder (*AD*), and Huntington's disease (*HD*) were examined using the motor impairment scale (MIS) of the quantified neurologic examination (QNE) developed for HD. Schizophrenics and affectives with tardive dyskinesia (*TD*), who were matched for severity of involuntary movement with HD patients, had significantly lower ratings of voluntary motor abnormalities on the MIS (P <.001). Schizophrenics with Parkinsonian signs (*PD*) had higher MIS scores, but they were still significantly lower (P <.005) than HD patients matched for involuntary movements. (Source: David et al. 1987, reprinted with permission.)

(TD). Patients with TD may have severe chorea but only modest impairment in voluntary movement (Crane 1973; David et al. 1987). Their voluntary movements are quick and accurate, their gait is narrowly based, they are able to tandem walk, and they do not suffer from dysarthria or dysphagia. When examined using the QNE, TD patients, matched with HD patients for the severity of their involuntary movements, had significantly lower scores than HD patients on the motor impairment scale (figure 2.4).

Finally, a number of investigators have reported that drugs affect chorea and voluntary movement in different ways (Nutt and Morgan 1983; Bassi et al. 1986; Koller and Trimble 1985). Among reports of experimental therapeutic studies, four measured the response of chorea and coordination separately. Chorea, but not coordination, improved in response to dopamine antagonists (haloperidol and transdihydrolisuride) and the anticholinergic agent scopolamine. One drug, tiapride, a dopamine-2 receptor antagonist, resulted in improvement in both chorea and motor speed and coordination (Deroover et al. 1984). As demonstrated by Nutt and Morgan, many of the contradictory outcomes of experimental therapeutic studies in Huntington's disease result from the failure to consider responses of involuntary and voluntary motor impairment separately.

Neuropathologic and Neurophysiologic Correlates

Given the differences between involuntary and voluntary movements in their relationships to duration of illness, in their correlations with other clinical variables, and in their responses to pharmacologic agents, it is reasonable to expect that they have different pathologies and pathophysiologies.

Studies of primates (reviewed by Alexander, DeLong, and Strick 1986) have demonstrated that, of the two major neostriatal nuclei, it is the putamen and not the caudate that receives fibers from the motor-related cortical areas. The putamen fires in relationship to several aspects of voluntary motor activity that are abnormal in HD: initiation of motor movements, motor speed, and persistence of motor activity. These findings can be demonstrated by electrophysiologic studies of the putamen in behaving primates and in ablation experiments.

Ablation of the putamen does not, however, result in involuntary movements. Chorea does result from the ablation of the subthalamic nucleus (STN) in humans and other primates (Whittier 1947; Carpenter, Whittier, and Mettler 1950). While neuronal loss is not consistently demonstrated in the STN in HD, wiring diagram models of the striatum (e.g., Penney and Young 1986; figure 5.4) suggest that the STN may be inhibited (i.e., neurophysiologically ablated) in HD as a result of increased inhibitory input to the STN from the globus pallidus.

Another possible explanation for chorea in HD (not necessarily incompatible with the one given above) comes from a consideration of the dopamine system in HD and tardive dyskinesia. Tardive dyskinesia is thought to result from prolonged blockade of the dopamine receptors in the striatum and their consequent supersensitivity (DeVeaugh-Geiss 1982). In HD there is also a relative excess of dopamine in the striatum, in this case a result of the preservation of dopamine input to the striatum in the face of decreasing numbers of dopamine receptors on the dying striatal neurons. In HD patients, chorea, but not voluntary motor impairment, responds to a blockade of striatal dopamine receptors by neuroleptic drugs.

The neural control of voluntary eye movements is somewhat different from that of other body parts, but the neostriatum (in this case the caudate) plays a central role and its destruction in HD is most likely the cause for abnormal saccades in early HD. Damage to the caudate nucleus interrupts the frontostriate circuit related to the control of eye movement. The direct result of this interruption is an alteration in voluntary eye movements in a way that is analogous to motor changes of other body parts: slowing, difficulty with initiation, and loss of persistence. In addition, the loss of striatal input to the superior colliculus may result in the loss of the patient's ability to voluntarily suppress reflexive saccades to sudden visual stimuli (Lasker et al. 1987).

Summary and Conclusions

The most easily observed motor abnormality in HD is chorea. However, it may be absent or overshadowed by other involuntary movements such as tremor or motor restlessness, bradykinesia, or clumsiness of voluntary motor movements. Voluntary and involuntary movement abnormalities are likely to be related to different subsystems within the basal ganglia and must be considered separately when studying pathophysiology and documenting the response to treatment.

3

The Cognitive Disorder

As the disease progresses the mind becomes more or less impaired, in many amounting to insanity.
—HUNTINGTON, 1872

Patients with Huntington's disease have cognitive deficits that begin early in the course of illness and worsen with time. These include trouble with memory, calculation, verbal fluency, visuospatial abilities, judgment, and speed of performance. Even when most formal tests of cognitive capacity show normal results, patients have great difficulty changing from one task to another (changing sets) and keeping track of several things at once (tracking multiple variables). Early in the illness, each of these aspects of cognition may be only mildly affected, but in sum they result in a loss of cognitive efficiency and interfere with function (Mayeux et al. 1986). HD patients have a dementia (i.e., a global cognitive decline in clear consciousness), but they do not have aphasia or agnosia and rarely apraxia, the cardinal features of the dementia of Alzheimer's disease. The dementia of HD is one of the subcortical dementias, characterized by a memory defect, cognitive slowing, apathy, and depression (McHugh and Folstein 1973; Albert, Feldman, and Willis 1974), but a sparing of the ability to comprehend and express language.

This chapter describes the dementia of HD as it is observed in three settings: at home and work, in the clinic, and during the performance of formal cognitive tests. It concludes with a discussion of the relationships between the cognitive deficits and the neural mechanisms that may underlie them.

Case Example: The Course of Cognitive Decline in One Patient

Dr. Matthews had a Ph.D. and taught at a state university. By age 35, he had been promoted to associate professor. At age 38, he became an advocate for students who were threatened with disciplinary action. At first, this seemed a natural outgrowth of an earlier interest in civil rights, but, as time passed, colleagues became puzzled by both Dr. Matthews' judgment of the merits of particular cases and the appropriateness of his tactics.

Dr. Matthews began to miss classes, his lectures became poorly organized, and fewer students took his courses. His wife became concerned and convinced him to seek psychotherapy.

After two years, the university administration became sufficiently concerned about Dr. Matthews' student advocacy activities to initiate disciplinary proceedings. Dr. Matthews defended himself vigorously, claiming unfair treatment, and hired a lawyer. Meanwhile, he voiced his complaints to anyone who would listen and demanded fewer course assignments so that he could write a book.

By this time, Dr. Matthews had mild choreic movements. Mrs. Matthews encouraged him to see a neurologist, who diagnosed HD. At the initial examination, Dr. Matthews' score on the Mini-Mental State Examination (MMSE) (Folstein, Folstein, and McHugh 1975), a cognitive screening test, was 30/30 and his full-scale intelligence quotient was 111 on the Wechsler Adult Intelligence Test (WAIS), with a verbal IQ of 120 and a performance IQ of 99. He denied illness and argued that his symptoms resulted from stress and an earlier automobile accident.

Sympathetic colleagues and Mrs. Matthews described the changes in Dr. Matthews' intellect. His talk had become more circumstantial and less fluent. It was irritating to wait for him to get to the point. He would sit for several hours preparing a lecture, but he spent the time shuffling papers, starting over, pacing about, and accomplishing little. At other times, he sat idle in his office. He said he was thinking about his book. At home, he stopped paying the bills and made poor judgments about household purchases.

Dr. Matthews finally accepted retirement from the university with full disability. Three years later, his MMSE score was 25/30, with four points deducted for calculation and one for recall of words. His full-scale IQ had dropped to 100, with a verbal IQ of 105 and a performance IQ of 85. He took less part in conversation, saying that the verbal exchanges occurred too quickly for him to gather his thoughts and make any timely remark. He still read for several hours a day and claimed to recall the content, but his discussion of a book was brief and superficial. At home he needed to be reminded of tasks that were not routine. One day, his wife left his lunch on a different shelf in the refrigerator and he could not find it.

Cognitive Impairment as It Presents at Home and at Work

Patients vary in the extent to which cognition declines early in the illness. Trouble with memory and the inability to organize and systematically execute a day's work usually occur early and are often the first symptoms with important functional consequences. A few patients can continue to work at intellectually demanding jobs well after the onset of motor signs. These are usually persons whose symptoms have begun later in life (after age 50), who had a high intellectual capacity before the illness, and whose jobs, while demanding a high level of performance, are thoroughly familiar to them from many years of experience.

Specific complaints vary from patient to patient, but concerns about short-term memory usually feature prominently. Homemakers forget to collect the children from school or overlook listed items they intended to buy at the supermarket. However, memory is rarely the only problem. Patients are less able to work under time pressure, move from one task to another, or initiate any activity. Some previously conscientious homemakers sit all day watching television, seemingly uninterested in their housekeeping. Those patients who are still motivated to keep house complain that everything takes longer, and they have difficulty getting from one task to the next or are unable to assemble all the materials needed for tasks that include several steps.

The most difficult jobs are those that require decisions for which there are no preexisting guidelines, self-initiated changes from one task to the next (such as secretarial work), arithmetic computations or number copying (bookkeeping or computer work), or visuomotor integrations (auto mechanics) (Fisher et al. 1983; Brandt and Butters 1986). Persons who work at repetitive jobs can often work longer into the illness, until motor problems cause job failure. Repetitive assembly line or other factory work may be easier, not only because of its lack of complexity, but also because others are involved in the task, so the patient does not have to initiate the task or move from one task to another unprompted.

Job failure can be precipitated by a promotion or change in job assignment. While patients can often continue to perform familiar tasks, it is extremely difficult for them to learn a new one, even if it is no more difficult than the one previously performed. At first, it may be difficult for the family or employer to understand these performance failures as the result of an illness. The condition is usually undiagnosed, and most employers and a surprising number of family members are unaware that the person is at risk for HD. The change in performance may be attributed to alcoholism (motor clumsiness is sometimes present) or may be interpreted as the attempt of a disgruntled employee to get back at the boss.

Eventually even HD patients who retain their motivation and whose involuntary movements are mild fail at their jobs because they lose the ability to perform quickly enough to complete the job. This can result from the combination of several mild motor and cognitive difficulties, but cognitive and motor speed and the failure to change to the next task play important roles. Functioning on the job may also be impaired by the patient's loss of judgment and frequent loss of temper at work. The loss of temper usually occurs when the patient is asked to hurry or to perform a task that has become too difficult. Small irritants that would previously have been overlooked can cause major outbursts.

After stopping work (either outside or in the home), many patients are unable to initiate activities for themselves, and they may resist attempts by others to organize activities for them. There are many notable exceptions, however. Some patients continue to drive and keep house long after motor impairment makes it dangerous for them to do so. Others busy themselves effectively with yard work or other aspects of home maintenance. A few are able to maintain enough concentration to read for a number of years. For the most part, however, family members report that the patient's days lack activity, except that initiated and maintained by others. Spouses are initially annoyed by this because they observe that the patients *can* perform, and they want more help from the patient with domestic activities. Patients asked to perform some tasks will forget or do the first task but not the others.

Patients also gradually decrease their participation in conversation (Gordon and Illes 1987). They find that they are not fluent enough to keep pace and that the topic has changed by the time they formulate a reply. Eventually it becomes difficult for them even to initiate speech, and their severe dysarthria discourages them from attempting to make themselves understood. By this stage, patients will also have difficulty understanding complex, multiple-step conversations and abstract topics.

Late in the illness, dementia is often quite severe, although one patient was known to keep a daily journal after 25 years of illness. For the most part, patients become mute after 15 years of illness, but, to the end of life, many watch television (and request channel changes at appropriate times), are able to comprehend simple statements and requests, recognize relatives, and retain enough sense of orientation to know when to expect visits (and enough sense of justice to be angry when no one appears). This is quite different from the dementia of Alzheimer's disease, in which patients eventually lose the ability to comprehend speech, misidentify even the closest relatives, and are completely disoriented.

The Detection of Cognitive Deficits in the Clinic

Cognition can be assessed in the clinical setting without the use of lengthy tests. This can be accomplished during history taking and with brief but formal tests of cognition.

The Assessment of Cognition while Taking a History

To obtain an accurate history, either at an initial evaluation or during the course of care of HD patients, it is important for the examiner to include a spouse or another informant in the process. This also allows the examiner to compare the patient's memory for remote and recent events of personal life with the spouse's memory for the same events. For example, the patient may turn to his spouse to provide information about dates of children's birth, employment, or episodes of depression. He may be vague in recalling signs or symptoms, particularly their duration and the circumstances surrounding them. During conversation, the patient may have difficulty finding words and offer little spontaneous speech. The paucity of conversation may be a sign of depression, but often it indicates cognitive slowing.

The Mini-Mental State Examination (MMSE)

To test cognition quickly during clinical examination, the MMSE (appendix 1) or some other structured cognitive screening test may be used to estimate the type and variety of cognitive deficit and to follow the patient longitudinally. In our experience, all patients show a gradual cognitive decline with time (figure 3.1). Nevertheless, they vary tremendously in the severity and rate of progression of their cognitive deficit (table 3.1). This variation is largely a function of the years of education. In a multiple regression analysis, education and duration of illness were equally strong predictors of the MMSE total score, with P values <.0001 (Folstein, unpublished data).

While failure on cognitive screening tests is associated with failure at work, successful test performance is not an accurate indicator of the patient's ability to work. Some patients who score in the normal range on the MMSE (and on IQ tests; see below) are unable to function at a job because of their difficulty in initiating and sustaining work and handling more complex tasks. Although the ability to perform on the MMSE is usually better than the actual functional capacity, the two are strongly correlated. MMSE scores are more closely

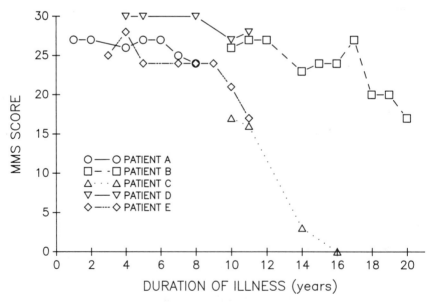

Figure 3.1. The change with time of the MMSE scores of five patients followed in the BHDP Research Clinic illustrates the variable rate of decline for cognition.

Table 3.1. Huntington's Disease Patients Grouped by Total MMSE Score and Duration of Illness

Duration of Illness	MMSE Total Score				
	26–30	21–25	16–20	10–15	<10
Range (years)	0–15	0–36	0–31	5–25	2–29
Mean (SD)	4.7 (4.0)	8.3 (6.8)	8.8 (6.8)	14.0 (6.9)	13.7 (6.0)
	(N = 41)	(N = 49)	(N = 35)	(N = 10)	(N = 46)

Note: For HD patients with scores on the MMSE within a given range, the duration of illness varied widely, although the mean duration of illness increased steadily as MMSE scores declined. Some of the variation was attributable to years of education (see text).

related to the ability to function at work and at home than is the duration of the illness (table 2.3; see also Brandt et al. 1984).

Performance on Individual MMSE Items

While scores on MMSE items all show a gradual decline over time, the rate of decline is not uniform from item to item. This can best be demonstrated by comparing HD patients with Alzheimer's disease (AD) patients, matched for overall MMSE scores (figure 3.2 *A,B,C;* see also Brandt, Folstein, and Folstein 1988). Individual items are discussed in the order in which performance becomes impaired, beginning with those affected early in the course of the illness.

Serial Sevens   The first item on the MMSE to be affected in HD patients is usually serial sevens, a task of calculation and concentration in which the patient is asked to start at 100 and subtract 7, repeating the process until five subtractions are performed. In the general population, performance on serial sevens is unrelated to education above the eighth grade level (Anthony et al. 1982), but it does appear from clinical experience to be less affected in persons who have worked in jobs requiring the frequent use of computation. Performance is significantly worse in HD than AD patients matched for MMSE total scores from 24 down to 10, at which level no HD patient scores any points on the item.

Recall of Three Words   The recall of three words following a brief distraction is affected early in the course, although not so severely as in AD. Most patients will usually recall one or two of the words, and many will remember all three. Again, there are exceptional patients who continue to perform normally on this and more difficult memory tasks, and whose memory is reported by family members to be unimpaired for many years after the onset of symptoms.

Orientation, Copying Figures   Somewhat later in the course of illness, the more difficult orientation items (such as the date and the floor of the clinic), will be missed. However, orientation is preserved better than in AD patients at the

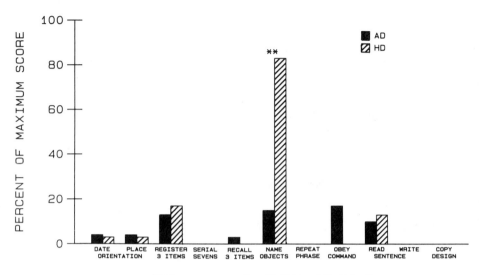

Figure 3.2. Patients with *HD* and Alzheimer's disease (*AD*), matched for total MMSE score, were compared on the individual MMSE items. Scores are expressed as percentages because not all items have the same total possible points. The serial sevens score dropped more quickly in HD, while memory and orientation were preserved relative to AD patients with the same total MMSE scores (*A, opposite top; B, opposite, bottom*). Most HD patients with very low MMSE scores could still name objects (*C, above*). Single asterisk indicates the difference is significant at P <.01; double asterisk indicates P <.001.
(Source: Brandt, Folstein and Folstein 1988, reprinted with permission.)

same MMSE level. About the same time, patients begin to have difficulty copying interlocking pentagons, another item that is performed poorly by normal subjects with less than an eighth-grade education. The failure is one of perception of shape and is unrelated to the severity of involuntary movements, as assessed by many observations of HD patients. HD patients who can adequately hold a pencil and execute the drawing make serious errors in the number of sides, number of angles, and position of the interlocking angles. They sometimes look at the example several times and attempt to correct their copy, realizing that it is incorrect but usually unable to see why.

Writing a Coherent Sentence   Some patients are able to write a sentence for as long as they can effectively move their hands. However, the sentences become shorter and less complex in construction. Other patients begin to fail at sentence

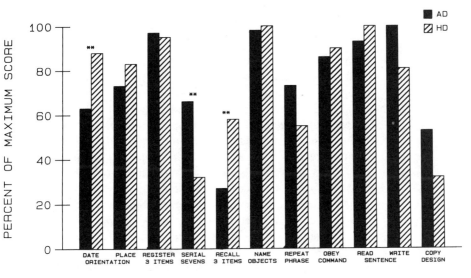

Fig. 3-2

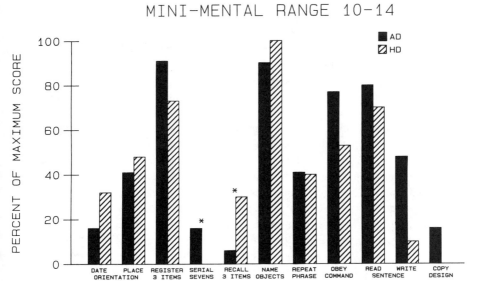

Fig. 3-2

construction after 10 years of illness. Most persons with MMSE scores below 14 are unable to write a sentence, usually because of cognitive failure but sometimes because of motor disability. In this regard, HD patients perform more poorly than AD patients.

Registration, Naming, Reading, and Easy Orientation Items   At moderate levels of dementia (MMSE 10–14), HD patients are at least partially oriented and retain the ability to register three words (repeat them after the examiner), name objects, and read a sentence. At more advanced stages, performance is so impaired by motor difficulties that only the items that require simple verbal utterances are successfully performed. Even patients with severe dysarthria can be understood if the examiner is expecting a limited range of responses. Some can spell the reply—letters are more easily understood than words. However, when the total MMSE score is as low as 1–4, orientation items, which can be successfully tested by speech alone, are mostly failed. Naming is the last skill lost. Even when patients have great difficulty in initiating speech, they can sometimes, with a great expenditure of energy, name simple objects such as a pen or a watch. This success gives them obvious pleasure.

A few of the items on the MMSE are difficult to interpret because of motor or education effects. The repetition of a phrase ("No if's, and's, or but's") appears to be related to dysarthria more than to dementia. Executing a three-stage command is impaired by a mixture of motor and cognitive deficits.

Intelligence Tests in Huntington's Disease

Full-scale IQ as measured by the Wechsler Adult Intelligence Scale (WAIS) drops modestly during the first years of illness, the performance scale accounting for most of the decline (Lyle and Gottesman 1977). As the illness progresses, scores continue to fall slightly, but patients rarely score in the mentally retarded range (below 70) until ten or more years after onset. Longitudinal data on a few individual patients demonstrate the gradual decline in IQ (figure 3.3).

The various subtests of the WAIS are not all equally affected (figure 3.4). Vocabulary (defining words) and information (general knowledge) are spared, more than other cognitive functions until late in the illness. Arithmetic (mental calculation), digit symbol (matching numbers with symbols as quickly as possible), picture arrangement (arranging pictures in a logical sequence), and digit span (repeating a series of numbers) are impaired early in the illness (Norton 1975; Butters et al. 1978; Josiassen et al. 1982). The vulnerability of these subtests makes sense in light of the clinical observations of impairments in memory, arithmetic, rapid performance of complex tasks, and sequential task performance.

This typical uneven pattern of performance on WAIS subtests is seen early in the illness, and led several investigators to explore using the WAIS pattern for

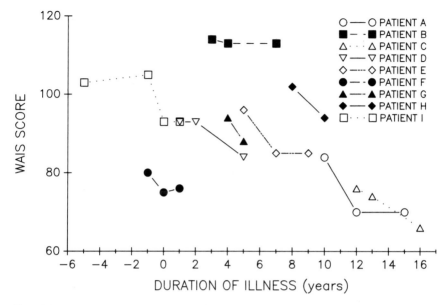

Figure 3.3. Intelligence, as measured by the Wechsler Adult Intelligence Scale (WAIS), declines as the illness progresses. However, in some patients the measured full-scale IQ is still above the mentally retarded range after twelve years of illness. This illustrates the difficulty in demonstrating the considerable cognitive deficits in HD with IQ tests.

presymptomatic testing (Lyle and Gottesman 1977; Josiassen et al. 1982; Strauss and Brandt 1986). However, because of the individual variability in premorbid subtest patterns, the WAIS is not a useful predictor of illness for individual cases despite consistent group differences between at-risk persons who later become affected and those who escape HD. It may be possible to utilize IQ tests longitudinally as indicators of onset among individual at-risk persons who are in long-term follow-up and who can thus serve as their own controls. A few at-risk persons have been tested repeatedly in BHDP projects during the presymptomatic period. Performance IQ dropped around the time of onset of barely detectable motor and cognitive symptoms.

IQ Tests in the Determination of Disability

It is important to stress that IQ tests are not useful in supporting a disability claim for patients with HD. At the time the patient has been forced to retire from work and is applying for Social Security Disability Insurance (SSDI), the IQ remains well above the cut-off score for designation as retarded (IQ of 70). IQ tests are often ordered by the SSDI claims investigators and, if the results are reported without a detailed explanation of the disparity between test perfor-

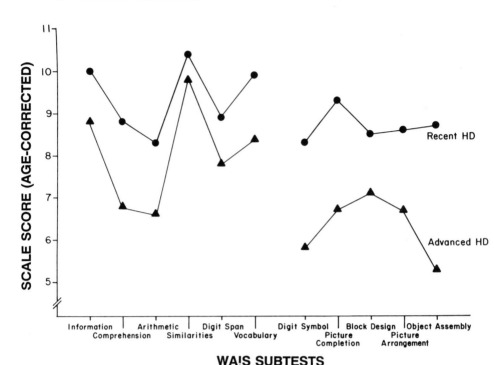

WAIS SUBTESTS

Figure 3.4. The nonverbal scale on the WAIS declines more quickly than the verbal scale. The verbal scale has a characteristic "sawtooth" pattern when measured early in the illness (circles) and after several years of illness (triangles).
(Source: Brandt et al. 1984, reprinted with permission.)

mance and functional capacity in a work setting, patients will probably be denied SSDI on the grounds that they are not demented. (Dementia is often the major justification for disability, since motor impairment is usually mild at the time patients are no longer able to hold a job.) IQ test results do not adequately reflect the dementia of HD; other tests of specific cognitive functions more accurately reflect the patient's loss of the capacity for gainful employment.

The Measurement of Specific Cognitive Deficits in Huntington's Disease

Memory Loss

Memory has been studied more than any other aspect of cognition in HD, and experiments have often contrasted the performance of HD patients with that of patients suffering from Korsakoff's syndrome or Alzheimer's disease. The pattern of memory and other cognitive deficits in HD varies depending on the severity of illness, which more recent studies have taken into account. Not all investigators use the same method of estimating disease duration or severity, making comparisons difficult. However, the bulk of evidence suggests that new memories can be adequately encoded, but the information cannot be recalled upon demand. Similarly, many old memories are retained but cannot be efficiently retrieved.

Early studies testing the learning of new material suggested that HD patients either were not adequately encoding (Buschke 1973; Weingartner, Caine, and Ebert 1979) or were not storing (e.g., Butters et al. 1976) new memories. More detailed analysis of their performance now suggests that memories are stored but cannot be retrieved at will (Wilson and Garron 1979; Caine et al. 1986). When recalling word lists, normal subjects usually remember the same words after a 2-minute delay as they remembered earlier after a 15-second delay, but HD patients often recall *different* words (ones they had not previously recalled) after the longer delay (Moss et al. 1986). Caine, Ebert, and Weingartner (1977) made this same observation, noting that HD patients would sometimes recall words the next day that they had not recalled during the testing session.

This phenomenon is occasionally reported by families and may account for their insistence, in the face of abnormal test results, that their affected relative has a normal memory. One spouse described a conversation among family members who were trying to recall the married name of another relative. No one succeeded and the topic was dropped. The patient, who was present but had not participated in the conversation, blurted out the relative's name about 30 minutes later.

Other observations also support the hypothesis that the memory deficit in HD is primarily a retrieval problem. HD patients accurately *recognize* recently presented verbal material that they were not able to *recall* when asked to recite the material without cues. This observation has been made now by several investigators using diverse testing paradigms (Albert, Butters, and Brandt 1981a, 1981b; Butters 1984; Martone et al. 1984; Moss et al. 1986; Butters, Wolfe, and Granholm 1986). Patients with an encoding deficit (as in Korsakoff's syndrome) do not perform better on recognition than on recall.

Similar observations have been made regarding remote memories. Caine et al. (1978) were able to improve HD patients' recall of their own personal histories by introducing a multiple-choice recognition task. Brandt (1985) studied long-term factual memory, or world knowledge, by asking HD patients first to recall the answers to such questions as "What is the largest planet in the solar system?" For the unanswered questions, the patients were asked if they had a feeling that they knew the answer. As in the normal control group, this feeling of knowing correlated well with their ability to recognize the correct answer on a multiple-choice test, supporting the hypothesis that remote memories were still present but could not be retrieved upon demand.

At least two studies (Albert, Butters, and Brandt 1981a; Brandt 1985) have shown that HD patients have equal difficulty with remote memories from all decades. That is, there is no memory gradient as seen in Korsakoff's syndrome, in which the most remote memories are spared, and there is a progressive fall-off of more recent memories.

The distinction between the encoding and the retrieval of verbal material is most clearly observed in HD patients who have been ill for only a few years and have relatively mild deficits in functional capacity, but similar patterns may be observed in patients with moderately advanced disease, even though the absolute level of performance is lower.

Most of the memory studies of HD patients have been limited to material presented verbally. However, one study by Moss et al. (1986) compared recognition memory for written words, colors, position of markers on a board, simple linear designs, and faces. Each test used the same paradigm, so test difficulty across categories of stimuli was comparable. The HD patients performed as well as normal controls *only* on the recognition of written words. Their recognition memory in all other test situations was severely impaired and did not differ from that of patients with Alzheimer's disease or Korsakoff's syndrome, suggesting that it is possible that verbal memory may be relatively spared in HD (Josiassen, Curry, and Mancall 1983). Alternatively, the general visuospatial deficits seen in HD (see below) may interfere with the testing of memory for nonverbal material.

Language

The language deficits measured in HD patients may also reflect retained verbal *recognition* memory coupled with impaired ability to search for and retrieve memories (*recall*). The ability to name objects (word recognition) is retained until it can no longer be tested because of severe dysarthria or mutism. Similarly, straightforward declarative speech can be comprehended (or recognized) by HD patients long after they become mute. However, the fluency of expressive language (or recall of words from memory) is severely affected early in the disease process.

In the FAS test of verbal fluency or word recall (Borkowski, Benton, and Spreen 1967), the patient is asked to say as many words as possible that begin with the letters *F*, *A*, and *S*. One minute is allowed for each letter. Quite early in the illness, HD patients score well below education-, sex-, and age-based norms. They say a few words and then fall silent even if prompted to continue the task, and they seldom remember additional words within the allowed minute. Later in the testing session, however, they may spontaneously mention some other words.

Poor performance on the FAS recall test is in sharp contrast to performance on the Boston Naming Test (BNT), a test of picture recognition (Butters et al. 1978). The BNT consists of a series of line drawings of common objects that patients are asked to name. Most HD patients usually achieve high scores, even in the advanced stages of illness, if points are not deducted for slow performance. The pattern of performances on the FAS and BNT is different from that seen in patients with Alzheimer's disease, whose fluency and picture recognition are equally and severely affected and whose errors on the two tasks are different (Kramer et al. 1988).

Attention and Concentration

HD patients have difficulty sustaining their performance on a wide variety of everyday tasks, both motor and cognitive, suggesting difficulties in concentration. Most tests of attention and concentration require additional cognitive skills, so they are difficult to measure in isolation. Over a wide range of tasks that require sustained concentration, such as mental arithmetic, digit-symbol (matching numbers with symbols that have been arbitrarily assigned to them), and reaction time, HD patients perform below the level expected for their overall cognitive ability.

Visuospatial Ability

Although patients usually do not have apraxia (as measured by their ability to dress themselves or mimic motor acts), their visuospatial skills are clearly abnormal, even early in the illness, when failures cannot be attributed to general cognitive decline or difficulties with motor coordination (Josiassen, Curry and Mancall 1983). Early deficits have been documented in the WAIS subtests measuring visuomotor skill, such as object assembly (jigsawlike puzzles) and block design (constructing a geometric pattern using colored cubes). In addition, deficits are detected in tests that do not require a motor act (Moses et al. 1981; Fedio et al. 1979). Fedio demonstrated this using the mosaic comparisons task. Subjects observed two grids of 9, 16, or 25 squares each and were asked to identify the one square that differed in the two grids. HD patients and some at-risk individuals performed more poorly than controls.

HD patients also have difficulty identifying their position in space, relative to some fixed point, if their own position in space is altered. In a study by Potegal (1971), patients observed a target and were then blindfolded and asked to point with a stylus to the position where the target had been. Patients were able to do this accurately unless they were moved one step to the side, after which they could no longer accurately localize the target. Potegal suggested that patients have difficulty in updating their position in space after a self-produced movement. He had previously identified this phenomenon in rats with caudate lesions. This deficit in updating egocentric spatial localization was also found by Brouwers et al. (1984), using different tasks. Their study also showed that patients with Alzheimer's disease retained egocentric spatial perception but lost the ability to perceive extrapersonal spatial relationships, tasks performed normally by HD patients in his sample. HD patients also have trouble with tasks involving left-right discriminations, especially when the positions are not consonant with their own, as, for example, in reading a road map (Fedio et al. 1979).

Changing Sets

Families often report that patients become rigid in their behavior, unable to change easily from one activity to another or to change their routines. This may be analogous to the great difficulty they have on cognitive tasks that require a change in set (Josiassen, Curry, and Mancall 1983; Fedio et al. 1979). On the Trail Making Test, part B, subjects are asked to connect the dots, but, instead of going directly from one number to another, they must alternate 1-A-2-B-3-C, etc. HD patients perform this much more slowly than would be expected from their score on part A, where they must connect only a series of numbers (Starkstein et al. 1988). The difficulty in changing sets is also demonstrated by the Wisconsin Card Sorting Test. Subjects are asked to sort cards by pattern, color, or number, but they must discern the rules only by the examiner saying "right" or "wrong" as the subject sorts the cards. Once the subject discerns the correct strategy, the examiner switches to a different one. HD patients quickly figure out the initial strategy but are not able to switch to others, persistently returning to the original one. In fact, any task that is complex, that requires frequent set changes, that uses more than one abstraction at once (Wexler 1979), or that uses rules not previously known to the subject (Fedio et al. 1979) will be difficult even for mildly affected HD patients.

Neuropathologic Correlates

The caudate nucleus, the striatal nucleus most severely and consistently affected in HD, is not connected to the motor cortex, but, instead, receives much of its cortical input from the frontal lobes, especially those areas serving to integrate cognitive functions. Therefore, it is not surprising that the cognitive functions affected in HD—the ability to plan and organize, verbal fluency, mental flexibility (changing sets), and some aspects of memory search and retrieval—are similar to those found in patients with frontal lobe disease (Stuss and Benson 1986).

Several investigators, using a variety of methods, have demonstrated the relationship of caudate pathology to cognitive changes in HD. Sax et al. (1983) reported that IQ and scores on the Wechsler Memory Scale were significantly correlated with caudate atrophy as measured by CT scan, and, furthermore, adding chorea to a multiple regression analysis did not add any significance to the variance accounted for once the cognitive variables were included. Bamford et al. (1986) reported similar findings. Richfield, Twyman, and Berent (1987) reported cognitive and behavioral abnormalities (but no motor signs) similar to those seen in HD in a patient with bilateral caudate damage. Starkstein et al. (1988) demonstrated a strong relationship between caudate atrophy as measured by CT and several cognitive tests (table 3.2). He found no signifi-

Table 3.2. Correlations between CT Measures and Neuropsychological Test Scores in 18 Huntington's Disease Patients

Test	BCR	BFR	FFR	4CSR
Mini-Mental Status				
R	−.49	.03	−.02	.06
P value	.002	NS	NS	NS
Symbol Digit Modalities (written)				
R	−.65	−.30	−.04	−.48
P value	.002	NS	NS	NS
Symbol Digit Modalities (oral)				
R	−.67	−.41	−.12	−.47
P value	.001	NS	NS	NS
Trails A (time)				
R	.72	.32	−.18	.43
P value	.001	NS	NS	NS
Trails B (time)				
R	.80	.48	−.29	.48
P value	.0001	NS	NS	NS

Source: Starkstein et al. in press. Reprinted with permission.

Note: Eighteen patients whose severity of illness varied were given CT scans and a series of cognitive tests. All the cognitive tests correlated highly with a measure of caudate atrophy (bicaudate ratio, BCR) but not at all with measures of cortical atrophy: frontal horn size as measured by bifrontal ratio (BFR), the size of the frontal fissure (frontal fissure ratio, FFR), and a sum of the size of four cortical sulci (4CSR).

cant correlation between scores on cognitive tests and CT measures of cortical atrophy.

Evidence is accumulating that cognitive features in HD are related specifically to dysfunction in the caudate nucleus and that the cognitive functions involved are those served by the prefrontal cortex, which provides the major cortical input to the caudate. The other subcortical dementias, such as those seen in Parkinson's disease (Mortimer et al. 1987), supranuclear palsy, and the dementia of frontal lobe disease (Taylor, Saint-Cyr, and Lang 1986; Salazar et al. 1986), have many features in common with the dementia of HD and also have neuropathologies that interrupt the connections between the prefrontal cortex and its output to the caudate nucleus (Geshwind 1965).

Summary and Conclusions

Patients with HD suffer a nonaphasic but nonetheless global dementia that affects many cognitive functions, including verbal fluency, cognitive speed, the retrieval of memories, the ability to persist at a task, and the ability to change cognitive sets. Studies of primates (reviewed by Alexander, DeLong, and Strick 1986) and human disease (reviewed by Stuss and Benson 1986) have demonstrated that these functions are served by those parts of the frontal lobe that provide the major cortical input to the caudate nucleus. In CT and PET studies of HD patients, measures of caudate atrophy, but not cortical measures, correlate with the severity of cognitive deficit.

4

The Emotional Disorder

In all the families, or nearly all in which the choreic taint exists,
the nervous temperament greatly preponderates.
—HUNTINGTON, 1872

In his description of hereditary chorea (1872), George Huntington noted that "the tendency to insanity, and sometimes that form of insanity which leads to suicide, is marked." For this reason, people with Huntington's disease have traditionally been cared for in psychiatric hospitals, and psychiatrists have published descriptions of the emotional and behavioral features of the disorder since the beginning of this century (e.g., Hamilton 1908). In their early study of HD families living along the eastern seaboard of the United States, Davenport and Muncey (1916) described changes in mood which they considered to be indistinguishable from manic-depressive illness. Minski and Guttmann (1938) reviewed the high rate of suicide.

During the 1950s and 1960s, reports suggested that schizophrenia was the most common psychiatric syndrome associated with HD (reviewed by Garron 1973) and that changes in mood were understandable responses to chronic illness. At this time, under the influence of Bleuler's ideas, the definition of schizophrenia was broadened to include any "psychotic" symptoms, and mood changes were seen as psychologically understandable in terms of the patient's situation and background. Such interpretations were based upon theoretical concepts rather than empirical study.

As psychiatric research emerged in the late 1960s and 1970s as an empirical, rather than theoretical, endeavor using specified diagnostic criteria, studies of psychiatric illness in HD patients (Dewhurst et al. 1969; Oliver 1970; Bolt 1970; Mattsson 1974b; McHugh and Folstein 1975; Folstein, Folstein, and McHugh 1979) again reported high rates of depression and occasional manic symptoms, along with evidence suggesting that these mood abnormalities resulted from the neuropathology of HD. At the same time, empirical research in the phenomenology, neuroscience, genetics, and pharmacology of psychiatric disorders supported the view that manic-depressive illness and schizophrenia, both biologically induced conditions, are separate disorders with different neurochemical abnormalities and treatments. In light of these findings, we systematically investigated the psychiatric features of HD in a representative sample and attempted to relate these psychiatric features to the genetic aspects of HD and to its neuroanatomic and neurochemical pathology.

This chapter includes a description of the psychiatric features of HD as seen at home, at work, and in the clinic. A discussion follows of the results of an epidemiologic study of HD carried out by the Baltimore Huntington's Disease Project, reporting the prevalence of the most common psychiatric syndromes in HD, their relationship to the course of illness, and their uneven distribution in families and ethnic groups. The chapter concludes with a discussion of some possible relationships of these psychiatric features to the neuropathology and neurochemistry of HD.

Case Example: The Psychiatric Disorder of One Patient

Mr. and Mrs. Crane operated a successful farm supply business. Despite Mr. Crane's modest education, he made sound business decisions and was locally renowned for his aptitude for figures. The couple was noted in the community for their charitable acts. When Mr. Crane was 45 years old, he suffered an episode of depression with loss of weight, poor concentration, pervasive feelings of inadequacy, and concerns that he might have broken the law. After about eight months he recovered without treatment. The next year he had another episode of depression, preceded on this occasion by a week of elevated mood accompanied by a sense of well-being and increased talk containing frequent sexual innuendos. During the week of elevated mood, he made several risky purchases for the business and sent a large check—much more than his usual contributions—to a radio ministry. The mood swings continued, and family members, well aware that in their family HD was usually preceded by "going off," encouraged Mr. Crane to seek medical advice, which he refused to do. His wife was able to convince him to sell the business.

At age 50, Mr. Crane was admitted to the Johns Hopkins psychiatric inpatient service following a suicide attempt, with delusions of guilt, psychomotor retardation, and history of a 10-pound weight loss. He had mild-to-moderate choreic movements and an MMSE score of 27/30. He was treated with a tricyclic antidepressant and discharged improved, to be followed in the HD clinic. He attended irregularly, and after a few months refused to take the prescribed medication. He was admitted the next year to the same unit after threatening to harm his wife. At this admission he was cheerful, talkative, and expansive, and had much more striking choreic movements. He was able to convince the house staff that he was without psychiatric symptoms, but the nurses recognized the extreme difference in his mental state compared with his prior admission. They overheard a telephone conversation in which he ordered his wife (with threats of bodily harm) to send a large sum of money to the same religious organization and to come get him out of hospital. He refused medication, but his expansiveness gradually lessened, and he was discharged.

Mr. Crane continued to refuse medical attention, and his mood for the most part remained elevated, irritable, and threatening over the next two years. His wife moved out of the house after he became sexually provocative to his daughter and her friends. The house became dirty, and Mr. Crane wandered about the community, causing fear by his inappropriate behavior. He tried repeatedly to get access to an automobile and continued to squander large sums of money.

He was finally arrested and taken to a state psychiatric hospital where he was committed. On the unit, with regular meals, clear unpleasant consequences to his sexual approaches, and an invariant, structured routine, he gained weight and behaved much better, gradually winning the affection of the staff. His wife arranged for appointment of a legal guardian to manage Mr. Crane's money and instituted divorce proceedings. About one year later, a new physician was appointed to the unit. Mr. Crane convinced the new doctor that his wife wanted him home, and agreed to attend the HD clinic regularly for care. Discharge plans were stopped after the doctor was contacted in rapid succession by the patient's wife, guardian, and the Johns Hopkins HD clinic social worker, each of whom described the patient's history of irrational and unpredictable behavior.

The Presentation of Psychiatric Disorder at Home and at Work

The initial symptoms of HD are extremely variable. They can be motor, cognitive, emotional/behavioral, or any combination of the three. Patients commonly exhibit psychiatric disorder several years before other symptoms begin. This type of presentation is reported in as many as half of the cases in some case series (Heathfield 1967; Mattsson 1974b). Common presenting emotional symptoms are depression, irritability, and apathy.

Patients may have episodes of low mood, accompanied by a loss of energy and decreased ability to concentrate, which come and go for several years before other HD symptoms begin. Some patients seek treatment from psychiatrists or other mental health professionals, while others do not. Families notice these depressions as periods of decreased participation in social activities, decreased sexual interest, failure to prepare meals, or lack of interest in household chores. Some patients begin to think that family or friends have lost interest in them or become suspicious about their motivations. While depression may sometimes be chronic, it usually passes in three to nine months, forgotten until it returns. At work, depression may be manifested by increased nervousness, late arrival, failure to show up for work, or an increased social distance between the patient and colleagues. Level of performance may be adequate, but more time may be required to complete assignments.

Other patients may become excessively irritable, either as part of a depression or in the presence of a euthymic mood. When irritability is not a symptom of depression, it usually persists and may gradually worsen over time. Symptoms vary from mild (occasional harsh words to family members or coworkers that are out of character for that individual) to severe (explosive, angry responses to chance remarks or imagined slights, prolonged verbal harangues, and physical aggression to persons and property). Irritable and aggressive outbursts are commonly precipitated when a patient attempts a task that has become overtaxing, either physically or mentally, when the patient's authority or judgment is challenged, when family members are unwilling or unable to meet what they perceive as selfish demands, or when there is noise and confusion in the household. Occasionally, these behaviors are severe enough to be socially disabling for HD patients. When they occur early in the illness in a person whose spouse is unaware of the risk for HD, irritability often results in a loss of job or divorce. Severely irritable and aggressive patients sometimes behave antisocially. Children in the household may be physically abused (or fear that they will be). There may be altercations in public places and inappropriate use of firearms. Arrest and incarceration or psychiatric hospitalization usually result (Oliver 1970; Bolt 1970).

Other patients become apathetic as an initial symptom of psychiatric disorder. If unemployed, they sit at home watching television, unmotivated to perform their usual household tasks even though they deny any mood change and are physically quite capable of performing them. If employed outside the home, apathetic patients often quit their jobs or are fired for failure to turn up. Previously serious students fail to begin assignments until the last minute or skip classes, spending their time alone or "hanging out" with friends.

Occasionally, the first symptoms are abnormal perceptions, particularly delusions or auditory hallucinations. These may be detected only by the patient's request that everyone stop talking (when no one is present), by an apparent response to voices, or an insistence that family members take precautions against some kind of danger.

Rarely, patients manifest abnormal sexual behavior. (Interestingly, Huntington's own paper mentions two cases of sexual impropriety: married men about 50 years of age who "never let an opportunity to flirt with a pretty girl go past unimproved.") Most often this occurs in the context of a manic episode, but sometimes women or men may become habitually sexually promiscuous early in the course of the illness, and some men are arrested for indecent exposure, public masturbation, or sexual approaches to children. These behaviors are unusual, but are extremely disruptive to family and social life when they occur.

As the illness becomes well developed, most psychiatric symptoms persist and often worsen, and others—especially irritability and apathy—may appear. Patients with chronic mania or aggression are major problems for the family and the community, and, if their symptoms are unresponsive to available social and psychopharmacologic management, such patients require long-term care in psychiatric facilities well before their motor disorder becomes incapacitating. Late in the course, some patients have fewer depressions, although others have obvious signs of depression until death. Irritability gradually worsens and may become manageable only when the patient's outbursts are rendered harmless by a severe motor impairment. Sexual activity usually diminishes over time, with impotence in men and loss of interest by both men and women, although a few patients continue to make sexual approaches to family members or nursing staff when they can no longer walk and can barely speak.

The Detection of Psychiatric Disorder in the Clinic

Obtaining Adequate Information

Patients with HD often minimize their current symptoms and may have difficulty recalling past illnesses. For these reasons, it can be hard to obtain an accurate account of psychiatric disorder without an additional informant. For example, a spouse may recall depressive episodes that the patient has forgotten, describe changes in appetite and sleep patterns, or report a diurnal variation of mood, all of which may be denied by the patient. Patients may deny being depressed, but spouses will report patients' statements that illustrate their low mood and feelings of worthlessness or guilt. Patients may deny hallucinations but repeatedly ask the spouses why people in the other room keep talking about them. Most patients deny or minimize the extent of their irritability and aggression, often because they are ashamed of it. Others request treatment.

Another cause of difficulty in detecting emotional symptoms is that their expression in patients with HD may be modified by other symptoms of the disease. It is especially difficult to differentiate depression from apathy or to detect depression when the patient can no longer express himself effectively. Again, another informant is helpful. Spouses learn to detect a mood change from changes in the patient's characteristic behavior, activity level, or facial expression. In the absence of a spouse or other informant with a close relationship with the patient, medical records may be helpful in documenting past psychiatric history, but adequate documentation of current mental state may be impossible.

Diagnostic Criteria and Methods

The criteria used by the BHDP Research Clinic to diagnose psychiatric disorder in HD are those specified in the current diagnostic manual, *DSM IIIR* (American Psychiatric Association 1987) for psychiatric disorders. The criteria for schizophrenia, mania, and major depression have demonstrated reliability, and their validity is based upon specificities of symptomatology, course of illness, and response to specific treatments in case series and population studies.

The criteria for the more common psychiatric syndromes observed in HD patients are included in appendix 2 and are described below as the conditions present in HD patients in the clinic. We made three modifications to the use of the criteria. First, *DSM IIIR* does not allow for the diagnosis of specific psychiatric syndromes in persons with preexisting brain disease. We do not follow that rule because it does not allow diagnostic distinctions that are important in pharmacologic treatment of psychiatric symptoms of HD patients. Second, for the diagnosis of major affective disorder, we require an episode of depression to have lasted for at least four weeks (*DSM IIIR* requires only two weeks), because reactive depression is common and we wish to avoid pharmacologic intervention unless the low mood persists. Finally, we reserve judgment about the nature of depressions that are associated in time with the diagnosis of HD, divorce, loss of employment, or the death of an immediate family member even if they have persisted for four weeks. Such depressions are often reactive and resolve with emotional support and without pharmacologic intervention. If they persist, we begin a trial of antidepressants.

Specific Psychiatric Syndromes Seen in HD

The descriptions of psychiatric syndromes as they present in the clinic are based on our own research and a longitudinal follow-up of many HD patients. The longitudinal follow-up provides a different perspective from the one gained from cross-sectional evaluations, because some conditions wax and wane and others appear only late in the course.

Major Affective Disorder   Depression is the most common psychiatric syndrome seen in HD early in the course. It is characterized by a dysphoric, low mood, a change in self-attitude with feelings of self-depreciation, hopelessness, and occasionally guilt and suicidal thoughts or actions and by vegetative signs such as loss of interest and energy, anhedonia, insomnia with early morning awakening, loss of appetite, and a diurnal variation of mood with dysphoria worse in the morning hours.

Not all patients have all these symptoms. Some episodes are mild, with only loss of interest, energy, and mild dysphoria. Others are so severe that patients have delusions of poverty or fatal illness such as cancer. Some delusions are related to HD: patients may believe that death from HD is imminent even though symptoms are mild; others may believe that they deserve their fate because of past misdeeds.

Some HD patients with major affective disorder have episodes of mania as well as depression. Frank mania with delusions of grandeur and flight of ideas is uncommon, but brief episodes of hypomania, sometimes lasting only a few days, are observed in about 10% of patients. Hypomania is characterized by increased activity level (frantic house cleaning, pacing about) and pressured speech. Both of these behaviors are uncommon in nonmanic HD patients, who tend to become sedentary and uncommunicative. Patients may believe that they have found the cure for HD (one recommended gin and tonic) and display a general cheerfulness uncharacteristic for them. Some patients have a return of sexual interest after a long period of anhedonia or impotence. Others insist on making large and inappropriate expenditures, such as buying a new car when they are no longer able to drive. They may make serious attempts to resume driving or flying an airplane, although they may not have done so for many years and are clearly physically unable.

Hypomanic spells can be difficult to appreciate on cross-sectional encounter unless the examiner asks the informant specific questions about mood: patients may appear only rather unrealistically cheerful. When such an elevated mood is observed in demented HD patients, it is often described as "vacuous euphoria." Because the spells are somewhat uncommon and short-lived, the chance of observing one at a scheduled clinic visit is fairly small. However, if the family is questioned systematically for mood changes, the history can be elicited. Affective syndromes, whether only depressive or depressive alternating with manic, occur episodically in HD patients, with average depressive spells lasting 6 months or less, but approximately 20% of patients have chronic depressions. Hypomanic spells are usually shorter, lasting days to weeks but, again, a few patients have prolonged hypomania.

Affective syndromes are most commonly seen early in the course of the illness. Based on retrospective data, we estimated that episodic depression began an average of five years before motor symptoms. We are now able to confirm prospectively that affective disorder may precede any motor signs among at-risk persons in long-term follow-up. A few persons with a 99% probability of having the HD gene (by genetic marker study) have developed clear affective disorder without even subtle motor signs. When HD patients' medical records were reviewed during the Maryland HD survey, several HD patients were found who had been treated with electroconvulsive therapy (ECT) for depression some years before the diagnosis of HD was suspected. This also suggests that affective disorder may appear several years before the neurologic signs can be appreciated.

Affective disorder is more common in patients whose onset of motor symptoms occurs later. In the representative sample of HD patients from the Maryland survey, HD patients with affective disorder had an average age at onset of motor symptoms of 43 years, compared with 39 years for those patients without affective disorder (Folstein et al. 1987). This observation appears to conflict with that of Bolt (1970) and Mattsson (1974b), who reported that HD patients who presented with psychiatric disorder had a relatively earlier onset. This number, however, included cases that began with "personality changes" such as apathy and irritability.

It is understandable that physicians and other health care professionals find depression a logical mental state for HD patients to experience. They are, after all, suffering from a progressive deterioration of mind and body, and are doomed to "living out the dying" (Wexler 1975). There are several reasons why the hypothesis that depression is explainable on psychological grounds is not adequate. First, reactive depressions do not usually include all the symptoms that define major depression, particularly the change in self-attitude and some of the vegetative signs. Fewer than half of HD patients ever have an episode of major depression. Second, the depressions often occur as the first manifestation of HD, several years before the onset of motor symptoms or the loss of cognitive function in persons who are unaware of or unconcerned with their risk for HD (first noted by Minski and Guttmann 1938). Third, in about 10% of patients, the periods of low mood alternate with hypomanic spells, certainly not an understandable reaction to HD (Folstein, Abbott et al. 1983; Folstein et al. 1987). Fourth, the depressions respond to the same pharmacologic treatments used to manage major depression in the general population. Finally, cases of depression and mania are not randomly distributed in the HD population. The prevalence is quite high in some HD kindreds (up to 75% of cases) and low in others, as described below (Folstein, Abbott et al. 1983; Folstein et al. 1984).

Schizophrenia   Schizophrenia is characterized by two main features. The first is delusions (i.e., fixed, idiosyncratic beliefs that the patient holds despite evidence to the contrary). Occasionally, patients with depression or mania have delusions, but they are usually congruent with their depressed mood and altered self-attitude (e.g., delusions of poverty, illness, or guilt). Schizophrenic delusions are unrelated to mood, and the patient often associates their onset with some chance occurrence in the environment. For example, a patient saw a car behind him and knew, therefore, that the police department was keeping track of his activities. Some patients derive delusions from hallucinations. One patient thought her daughter poisoned her food after hearing voices telling her so. Another heard voices telling him that evil forces were trying to harm his family.

The second main feature of schizophrenia is auditory hallucinations. These vary widely in type, but two or more voices talking to each other or one voice giving a running commentary on the patient's activity are particularly characteristic of schizophrenia. The voices are usually vivid and clearly heard, perceived as coming from somewhere outside the head, and patients will often act upon the commands of the voices. Other kinds of hallucinations, tactile or visual, can be observed in addition to other symptoms such as thought broadcasting, thought insertion and withdrawal, and a disorder of the form of thought.

Most schizophrenic patients also have so-called negative symptoms such as loss of initiative, blunted affect, and failure to maintain personal relationships. These negative symptoms are quite common in HD patients. However, negative symptoms alone are not sufficient to diagnose schizophrenia and may occur in the context of many brain diseases.

Patients with HD do not always volunteer that they have delusions or hallucinations. They may be guarded and hostile or fearful, unwilling to provide any information or allow themselves to be examined. Family members will usually report behaviors suggesting the presence of abnormal perceptions. One patient asked a trusted friend why the people upstairs kept talking about her. Another refused to let his wife leave the house, insisting that voices had told him that someone would kill her if she left.

At the BHDP clinic, we have diagnosed schizophrenia in ten HD patients over 8 years. Not all were Maryland residents whose illness was present at the time of the survey, so there are fewer in the prevalence sample to be described below. Their ages at onset ranged from 15 to 44 years. Only one had an onset of motor symptoms after age 40. The patients could be divided into three groups. The two adolescents had delusions and hallucinations mixed with severe depressive symptoms and were resistant to pharmacologic treatment. Four patients with onset in adult life developed a variety of schizophrenic symptoms early in the course (e.g., delusions that a monitoring device was placed in his head; numerous voices commenting on his behavior). In two of these four cases, schizophrenic symptoms were present 10 years before abnormal movements were documented. In all cases, the symptoms were sensitive to phenothiazines, and in two cases followed longitudinally the symptoms eventually abated and required no further treatment. Three additional patients developed delusions and hallucinations about 10 or 12 years after the onset of the illness. These patients complained of various abnormal perceptions—such as tactile, visual, and auditory hallucinations—which were relieved in two cases by rather large doses of neuroleptics.

Another small group of patients have no delusions or hallucinations but have some of the subsidiary features of schizophrenia, such as thought disorder, suspiciousness of the motivations of others, hoarding of unneeded objects, and other peculiar behaviors. We excluded these patients from the diagnosis.

More commonly, patients with HD have the so-called negative symptoms of schizophrenia: apathy and a coarsening of personality and personal relationships. If not cared for, HD patients frequently become disheveled in their personal appearance and fail to maintain a clean living environment. During the Maryland HD survey, the psychiatric case notes were reviewed for many HD patients who had been diagnosed as schizophrenic during an admission to a psychiatric hospital. It is these negative symptoms that seem to be the reason for the diagnosis. Examiners making the diagnosis describe the patients' apathy and disconnectedness and comment on the absence of hallucinations and delusions. The diagnosis was primarily made without the benefit of an informant who knew the family history.

Irritability   Many patients with HD become irritable at some time during the course of the illness, and a few are aggressive. These behaviors, along with apathy and increasingly self-centered attitudes and behavior, are often lumped together in the HD literature as "personality change."

Regardless of its severity, irritability in HD has two general qualities: first, it is precipitated by some environmental event that previously would not have provoked as much response; and second, the severity and the duration of the irritable response are far out of proportion to the precipitant (Burns et al. in preparation). In the clinic, irritability is rarely observed unless the patient is delusional or has been coerced by his family into seeking treatment against his will. Most patients deny irritability, and it may be elicited only when the spouse is interviewed independently. The spouse may be afraid of the consequences of reporting irritability and aggression while in the patient's presence.

Irritability and aggression are more common in patients who have had these traits lifelong. They become exaggerated during illness. Irritability may also occur in patients without a prior history of a short temper. These patients are more likely to feel remorse about their inability to control their tempers.

Anxiety   Anxiety is a general feeling of tension and unrest, excessive worrying, and rumination about possible but often ill-defined trouble. Anxious persons may have sweaty palms and a wide-eyed, pained expression. HD patients may be anxious in the context of a depressive syndrome, but anxiety also appears in relation to events occurring in their environments. This diagnosis did not occur very often in our survey of psychiatric disorders in HD, probably because our methods of detection were not adequate. Nevertheless, clinicians who care for HD patients observe that they are excessively susceptible to anxiety regardless of other psychiatric syndromes that may be present.

Anxiety is easily detected in the clinic, a situation that is anxiety-provoking in the extreme for HD patients because it represents a concrete reminder of their fatal illness. They have sweaty palms, blood pressure that is higher than their internist reports, and choreiform movements more severe than those reported to occur at home. Evidence for anxiety can also be elicited during history taking. Patients report that they become extremely anxious at work, sometimes to the point of panic, when they cannot organize previously routine tasks. But anxiety is not always related to failures in performance. Families say that patients become overwhelmingly anxious about minor issues: "Why are you so late getting home?" "What should I wear?" "Should I accept the invitation?" "What if the weather is bad tomorrow?" or "Why must I bathe in the morning today?"

Sexual Behavior   Sexual behavior in HD has not been studied systematically, although it is of importance for two reasons. First, persons who later go on to have HD have more children than do their sibs who never develop the disease (Reed and Neel 1959; Marx 1973; Mattsson 1974b). This issue is discussed in chapter 7. The increase is accounted for by females with HD. Fewer males marry and have about the same number or fewer children than do their un-affected brothers. Second, clinical accounts of HD in the literature often describe individuals with HD who had abnormal or unacceptable sexual behaviors, (e.g., Bolt 1970; Oliver 1970) but the prevalence of this behavior in the HD population has never been studied.

In the BHDP research clinic, abnormal sexual behavior is usually reported in the context of legal difficulties with which the family requests assistance. For example, the patient's family may request a letter stating that the patient is ill to present at court in an attempt to quash charges of indecent exposure. Although sexual abuse of children by male HD patients is reported, the BHDP clinic has never had such a case. However, a few at-risk persons have reported being abused by their unaffected parent. Rarely, one of our patients has become sexually provocative to his children, and the mother has moved out or had the patient hospitalized.

The most common sexual complaint in the clinic is impotence in affected males. Commonly, after about 5 years of illness, males report impotence, even if they have not been treated with neuroleptic medication. Occasionally, a wife complains of rough sexual treatment or what she considers inappropriate or excessive sexual demands. This is hard to evaluate because the patient's changed behavior has often damaged the marital relationship to the extent that the spouse has lost sexual interest in the patient. Male spouses do not usually have complaints about an affected wife's sexual behavior, but they may comment that she accepts sexual activity but seems uninterested.

Alcoholism   There is a belief among families and some professionals (e.g., Chandler, Reed, and DeJong 1960) that patients with HD have a high rate of alcoholism. We did not find an excess of alcoholism in two separate investigations of HD patients in Maryland (King 1985; Folstein et al. 1986), nor did Bolt in Scotland (1970). In the survey of HD in Maryland (table 4.2 below), the rate of alcoholism was 15.6%, the same as that found in a concurrent community survey (Robins et al. 1984). However, we were not confident that our questions about the use of alcohol were sufficiently thorough. Therefore, in a second study, we systematically interviewed spouses of a representative subsample of the survey population specifically about alcohol use (King 1985). Before the onset of HD, approximately 16.7% of patients were heavy drinkers, about the same proportion we found in the original HD survey. After the onset of symptoms of HD, most drinkers voluntarily stopped, stating that they could no longer hold their liquor. Only 3 of our approximately 300 patients had serious consequences of alcoholism. One died in a fire that started accidentally during a solitary drinking bout, another was court ordered to give up his car and relinquish control of his financial assets because of drinking, and a third was hospitalized in long-term care because of consequences of alcoholism. Alcoholism is particularly troublesome in HD patients. Because their judgment is doubly impaired when they are drinking, by HD and by intoxication, their behavior can be extremely threatening and sometimes dangerously aggressive.

The Use of Tobacco   We have not systematically surveyed the use of tobacco among our patients. Many of them continue to smoke well after it has become unsafe because of their choreic movements and poor coordination. It is difficult to persuade HD patients to give up smoking, as it is with most smokers, and many continue until they no longer have access to cigarettes.

The Distribution of Psychiatric Disorder in Huntington's Disease

The Prevalence of Psychiatric Disorder in the HD Population

A major clinical research effort of the BHDP in the first 3 years of its existence was a systematic survey of HD in Maryland. One of our goals was to describe and estimate the prevalence of psychiatric disorder in a representative HD population. In previous surveys, patient samples were biased by referral to a psychiatric hospital (e.g., Dewhurst et al. 1969; Bickford and Ellison 1953; Minski and Guttmann 1938), did not use modern or systematic methods for making a psychiatric diagnosis (Chandler, Reed, and DeJong 1960; Wallace 1972), or had been forced to rely mainly on data from case notes with only a few direct interviews (Mattsson 1974b).

We were interested in this issue for several reasons. At the time the Maryland HD survey was undertaken, the prevailing view among clinicians and neuro-scientists was that HD might serve as a biologic model for schizophrenia. We were not convinced that schizophrenia was at all common among HD patients (McHugh and Folstein 1975), but a representative population study was needed to test the hypothesis systematically. Because of the view that HD patients were schizophrenic, many were being given pharmacologic treatments for schizo-phrenia but not for depression, which in our clinical experience with HD patients was more common (Folstein, Folstein, and McHugh 1979). Finally, we hoped that a clear delineation of the psychiatric features of individual patients, combined with studies of their brains, might provide clues to the pathophysiology of these psychiatric syndromes in the general population.

In the Maryland HD survey, we attempted to find and examine every HD patient who was symptomatic and living in Maryland on the last national census day, 1 April 1980. In such a survey, patients are seen at various stages of illness, and it is possible to state only what symptoms and syndromes have occurred in an individual patient up to the time of the survey. This means that psychiatric conditions that tend to occur early in the course of HD will be accurately counted, but those seen only late in the course will be underrepre-sented because not all the patients in the survey will have been observed through the entire course of their illness. In fact, most psychiatric disorders occur fairly early in the disease process, but we have noticed—having now followed some patients for up to 10 years—that schizophrenic syndromes

Table 4.1. Distribution of Psychiatric Disorder in Black and White Huntington's Disease Patients Ascertained in a Maryland Survey

DSM III Diagnosis	Number (%) of Subjects with Diagnosis[a]					
	Blacks		Whites		Total	
None	23	(46)	33	(24.3)	56	(30.1)[b]
Affective disorder	5	(10)	56	(41.2)	61	(32.8)[b]
Dysthymic disorder	5	(10)	4	(2.9)	9	(4.8)
Intermittent explosive disorder	10	(20)	47	(36.4)	57	(30.6)[b]
Alcoholism	9	(18)	20	(14.7)	29	(15.6)
Schizophrenia	1	(2)	7	(5.2)	8	(5.9)
Antisocial personality	5	(10)	6	(4.4)	11	(5.9)
Other	4	(8)	15	(11.0)	19	(10.2)
	(N = 50)		(N = 136)		(N = 186)	

Source: Folstein et al. 1987
[a]Totals exceed the number of patients because some patients met criteria for more than one DSM III diagnosis.
[b]Racial difference in proportions significant at P <.05.

occasionally appear for the first time late in the course. Therefore, their prevalence is probably slightly underestimated in the figures presented in table 4.1.

The most common condition we found in patients with HD was major affective disorder, followed closely by intermittent irritability approximating the condition known as intermittent explosive disorder. Schizophrenia was uncommon but was more common than expected from general population data. Alcoholism was found at the same rate as in the general population.

The BHDP survey is the only population-based study of HD that has included a systematic psychiatric evaluation, using personal interviews and standard diagnostic criteria. Therefore, it is not possible to provide exact comparisons with other studies. However, the studies of Bolt in Scotland, Oliver in England, and Mattsson in Sweden were based on total population samples and included some personal psychiatric interviews. Mattsson used broader criteria for schizophrenia than the BHDP study. Oliver reported symptoms rather than diagnoses but gave many useful case examples. The prevalence rates of psychiatric disorder, as estimated from their reported data, are summarized in table 4.2. The most common symptoms reported by these studies were disturbances in mood and "personality change," which in most cases was characterized by increased irritability and aggression.

The Differences between Families and between Races

Since the early twentieth century (Davenport and Muncey 1916), clinicians who have systematically examined HD patients and families have been struck

Table 4.2. Distribution of Psychiatric Disorder in Population Studies of Huntington's Disease that Included Psychiatric Interviews and Diagnoses

	Study		
Disorder	Bolt 1970	Oliver 1970	Mattsson 1974
Depression	25%	approx. 25%	16%[a]
Suicide threats and attempts	1%	4%	32%
Elation and grandiosity	5%	2%	not reported
Irritability and aggression	50%	35%	20%[a]
Schizophrenia	4%	0%	12%[a,b]
Sexual abnormalities	6%	6%	not reported
Alcoholism	4%	not reported	not reported

Note: In some cases, percentages are estimated from data.
[a]Includes only presenting psychiatric symptoms, not those that appeared later in the course of the illness.
[b]Includes patients called schizophrenic on the basis of "thought disorder" and "disturbances in self."

by differences between families. Most such observations have been made with respect to the age at the onset of symptoms, but a few studies considered motor abnormalities and emotional symptoms (reviewed by Folstein et al. 1984). Psychiatrists have repeatedly observed clustering of the two major psychiatric syndromes—affective disorder and schizophrenia—in certain HD families. The BHDP reported both family differences (Folstein, Abbott et al. 1983) and racial differences (Folstein et al. 1987) in the prevalence of affective disorder associated with HD.

Familial Aggregation of Major Affective Disorder   In the study of HD and affective disorder in families, we ascertained five families through a proband with HD and no psychiatric disorders except dementia, and five families through a proband who had both HD and bipolar affective disorder (episodes of both depression and mania). We chose bipolar probands to decrease the chances of choosing a proband who had a reactive depression. We obtained information on affected family members, unaffected relatives, the probands' spouses, and the spouses' siblings. As shown in table 4.3, the affected family members of the probands with both HD and affective disorder were also likely to have both disorders, whereas the family members of probands with HD alone were likely to have HD without associated major affective disorder.

Racial Differences in the Rate of Major Affective Disorder   The unexpected finding of 61 black HD patients in the Maryland survey provided the opportunity to compare the rate of psychiatric disorder in blacks and whites with HD (Folstein et al. 1987). Again unexpectedly, blacks rarely had major affective disorder

Table 4.3. Affective Disorder in Affected Relatives of Huntington's Disease Probands with and without Affective Disorder

Affective Disorder in Relatives with HD	Affective Disorder in Proband	
	Present	Absent
Present	20	5
Absent	3	18

Source: Folstein et al. 1983b
Note: $\chi^2 = 19.7$, P <0.001

and had less psychiatric disorder overall than did their white counterparts. Blacks also had an earlier average age at onset of symptoms and more often had the rigid akinetic form of HD, even when symptoms began during adult life.

Possible Neuropathologic and Neurochemical Correlates of the Psychiatric Syndromes Associated with Huntington's Disease

Numerous psychiatric syndromes can be delineated in HD patients. Some patients have more than one, being at once anxious, irritable, and subject to episodes of depression and hypomania. Occasional patients have a depressive syndrome early in the course and develop delusions and hallucinations later. This might seem to render the syndromes meaningless or at best nonspecific. However, if we consider that several brain areas and multiple neurochemical systems converge in the neostriatum, this multiplicity of psychiatric syndromes is not unexpected. As discussed in chapters 2 and 3, the motor and cognitive symptoms are similarly multiple.

Piecing together evidence from a variety of sources, one can make a few hypotheses about the neuroanatomic and neurochemical correlates of some of the emotional and perceptual abnormalities seen in HD. Given that major affective disorder occurs early in the illness, sometimes several years before other symptoms begin, it is likely to be related to changes in the medial anterior caudate (Folstein and Folstein 1987), since this part of the striatum is the first to show neuronal loss in HD (Vonsattel et al. 1985). This hypothesis is also supported by the fact that the medial anterior caudate receives considerable input from the limbic cortex, the part of the brain most likely to be directly related to emotional function (Gerfen 1984; Nauta 1986). In addition, affective disorder is commonly seen in patients with a variety of lesions of the basal ganglia (Folstein, Robinson et al. 1985; Starkstein, Robinson and Price 1987; Starkstein, Boston and Robinson 1988; Starkstein, Robinson et al. 1988; Trautner et al. 1988). Why all HD patients do not have affective disorder is not clear but could be related to a variation in patterns of neuropathologic change or to differences in vulnerability to affective disorder. For example, affective symptoms are unusual in blacks, who appear on limited evidence to have less caudate atrophy and more involvement of the motor-related substantia nigra compacta (Zweig et al. in press).

The ventral striatum and nucleus accumbens, often implicated in schizophrenia, are affected late in HD, except in juvenile-onset patients, in whom some pathologists report these ventral areas to be more severely affected. This may be consistent with the pattern of occurrence of schizophrenia in HD, which, as discussed above, may be more frequent late in the illness in adult-onset patients and is seen early in the illness in patients with juvenile onset.

Anxiety is extremely common in HD patients, and is probably present, to some extent, in all of them. This clinical finding may result from the connection between the benzodiazepine receptor and the γ-aminobutyric acid (GABA) receptor in the striatum and its major output target, the globus pallidus. Both GABA and GABA receptors are lost in the striatum in HD, and the GABA input to the globus pallidus from the striatum is likewise decreased. If the benzodiazepine receptor is related to human anxiety, its extreme disruption in HD may be the reason for the pervasive finding of anxiety in HD patients.

Summary and Conclusions

The emotional symptoms of HD cause considerable suffering to the patient and the family. Early in the course of illness they are the major cause for concern. Therefore, the emotional symptoms and syndromes need to be clearly delineated in individual patients so that appropriate treatment can be provided (as discussed in chapter 9).

It is understandable that physicians and other health-care professionals find depression, anxiety, and even irritability logical feelings for HD patients to have. Many of the emotional symptoms, however, appear to be a consequence of the neuropathology in HD and must be taken into account when considering the pathophysiology of HD and the functioning of the striatal system.

II

BASIC AND CLINICAL RESEARCH

5

Neuroscience

I know nothing of its pathology.
—HUNTINGTON, 1872

Huntington's disease is primarily a disease of the basal ganglia. Traditionally the basal ganglia have been conceived as influencing the output of the motor cortex. However, the clinical features of HD are not limited to the impairment of motor function but include a triad of motor, cognitive, and emotional abnormalities. Although the motor dysfunctions of HD have been attributed to pathology in the basal ganglia, the cognitive and emotional disorders have been thought to result from disease in other parts of the brain or have been explained as psychological reactions. As described in the preceding chapters, these are not adequate explanations. A variety of studies suggest that the cognitive and some of the emotional disorders as well as the motor abnormalities in HD are likely related to basal ganglia disease and thus suggest a wider role for the basal ganglia.

These clinical inferences have been supported and clarified in the last decade by anatomic, chemical, and physiologic studies of nonhuman primates and other mammals. These studies have demonstrated that the basal ganglia are involved not only in motor function but also in cognitive and emotional functions (reviewed by Alexander, DeLong, and Strick 1986). The clarification of the normal structure and function of the basal ganglia has not only supported the view that the triad of clinical features in HD is consistent with basal ganglia disease but also begun to suggest ways in which the particular basal ganglia pathology seen in HD may result in the signs and symptoms.

This chapter first summarizes our current understanding of the normal anatomy, chemistry, and function of the basal ganglia, then describes how these are altered in HD, and finally presents some current ideas about how these alterations lead to the clinical features of HD. Because the case example is more easily understood after the normal anatomy of the basal ganglia has been explained, it is presented at the end of that section.

The Normal Structure and Function of the Corpus Striatum

Gross Anatomy

The basal ganglia are comprised of several subcortical nuclei: the striatum, the globus pallidus, the substantia nigra, and the subthalamic nucleus. The striatum and the globus pallidus (or the pallidum) (figures 5.1, 5.2) are consistently affected in HD. The striatum and the pallidum are each comprised of a group of nuclei that are similar in microscopic structure, neurochemistry, and relationships to other brain structures (figure 5.3). The striatum, the "input center" for the basal ganglia, is composed of the caudate nucleus, putamen, and ventral striatum, which includes the nucleus accumbens and outer parts of the olfactory tubercle and adjacent areas. The pallidum, which receives the output from the striatum, is composed of the globus pallidus (lateral and medial segments) and the ventral pallidum, which includes parts of areas previously designated as lateral preoptic area and substantia innominata. These ventral areas have only recently been included in the definition of the striatum and pallidum, based on their similarities to the areas traditionally included (Heimer and Wilson 1975).

The striatum sends its output not only to the pallidum but also to the pars reticularis of the substantia nigra. The substantia nigra is actually two quite separate structures, the pars compacta (SNc, a group of dopamine-using neurons that sends fibers to the striatum) and the pars reticularis (SNr), which is similar in microscopic structure, neurochemistry, and connections to the medial pallidum and should be included as part of the pallidum (DeLong and Georgopoulos 1979; Nauta 1979). This text will refer to the two together as the pallidum-SNr.

In summary, the brain areas most prominently and consistently affected in HD have several different names, based on their shapes and on earlier concepts of their origins and functional relationships. However, they include only two basic neuron groups, the striatum, which is the input center of the basal ganglia, and the pallidum-SNr, the major recipient of its output.

Microscopic Anatomy

The nuclei within each of these two neuron groups have a similar microscopic anatomy. The striatal nuclei have two major neuronal types, spiny and aspiny, which are further subdivided according to size and other anatomic features (Pasik, Pasik, and DiFiglia 1976; DiFiglia, Pasik, and Pasik 1976, 1980). The spiny neurons are abundant (making up about 90% of the neurons in human striatum) and are the major output neurons, sending their axons to the pallidum-SNr. The aspiny neurons, much less common, are local circuit or interneurons with shorter axons that provide communication among the various incoming fibers and between striatal neurons (Graveland, Williams, and DiFiglia 1985a).

The most abundant neuron in the pallidum-SNr has a large cell body with a variety of dendritic types. Dendrites from one pallidal neuron synapse with

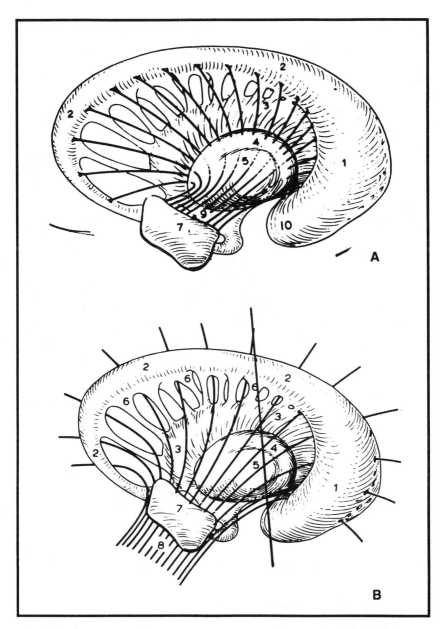

Figure 5.1. A simplified model of the basal ganglia is shown in the midsagittal plane, looking medial to lateral, (*A* and *B*). The caudate (*1* = head, *2* = body), putamen (*3*), and nucleus acumbens (*10*) can be seen to form one continuous structure, artificially separated by fibers of the corticospinal tract, the internal capsule (*8*, in *B*). The lateral globus pallidus (*4*), the medial globus (*5*), and substantia nigra (*7*) receive the output from the caudate and putamen through the striato-pallidal tract indicated by connecting lines, *9* in *A*). (Adapted from Gebbink, 1968, with permission.)

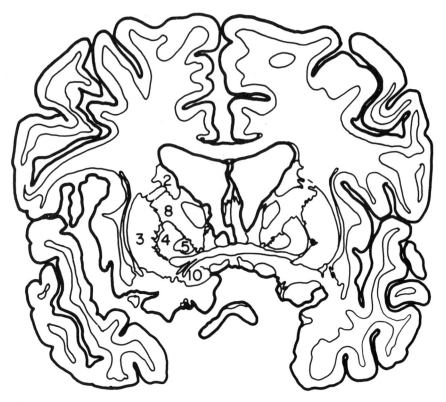

Figure 5.2. This line drawing of a human brain shows the same structures as figure 5.1, but viewed from the front in coronal section (cut at the line indicated on 5.1*B*). This view is often used in neuroanatomy texts. The basal ganglia structures are labelled using the same numbers as in fig. 5.1.
(Adapted from Nauta and Feritag, 1986, used with permission.)

many axon branches coming from the neostriatal spiny neurons. There are also some small interneurons in the lateral segment of the pallidum which are rarely seen in the medial pallidum (DiFiglia, Pasik, and Pasik 1982).

Fiber Connections of the Corpus Striatum

The Cortico-Striato-Pallido-Thalamo-Cortical Circuits   The striatum and the pallidum-SNr constitute two segments of a major cortical-subcortical circuit that begins and ends in the neocortex (figures 5.4, 5.5) (Graybiel and Ragsdale 1979). The circuit begins in neurons from diverse parts of the neocortex which send their axons to the striatum. These fibers synapse with various striatal neurons. Striatal spiny neurons send axons to the pallidum-SNr. These synapse with dendrites of the fusiform neurons of the pallidum, the axons of which go to particular

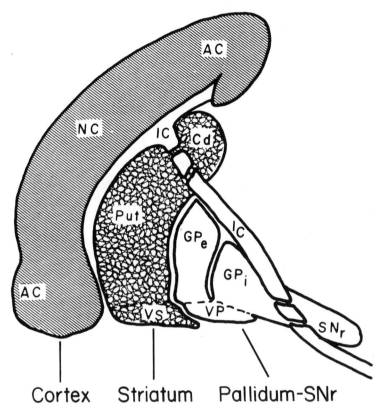

Cortex   Striatum   Pallidum-SNr

Figure 5.3. This drawing emphasizes the unity of each set of basal ganglia nuclei and their accidental separation by the internal capsule. *NC:* neocortex; *AC:* allocortex; *Cd:* caudate; *Put:* putamen; *VS:*ventral striatum; *GPe:* globus pallidus externa; *GPi:* globus pallidus interna; *VP:* ventral pallidum; *SN_r:* substantia nigra pars reticularis. (Source: Nauta 1986, reprinted with permission.)

nuclei of the thalamus. Thalamic fibers return to the cortex, but to more restricted areas than those from which the circuit originated.

In the past, it was generally believed that the striatum integrated the input coming from various parts of the cortex (i.e., mixed them together) and funneled the newly organized information back to the cortex via the ventrolateral thalamus. Recent anatomic and physiologic studies challenge this view. These studies suggest that the information coming into the striatum from different cortical areas remains generally anatomically segregated throughout the circuit.

Five major cortical-subcortical circuits have been proposed (figure 5.4), each of which travels to particular and separate areas of the striatum, pallidum-

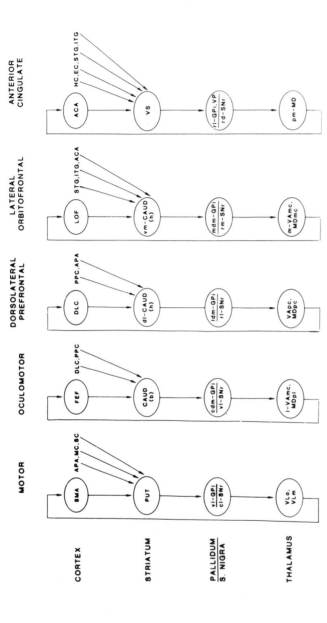

Figure 5.4. The five parallel corticostriate circuits that have been defined to date. Each circuit engages specific regions of the cerebral *cortex*, *striatum*, *pallidum*, *substantia nigra*, and *thalamus*, and each serves a relatively specified function. *ACA*: anterior cingulate area; *APA*: arcuate premotor area; *CAUD*: caudate, (*b*) body (*h*) head; *DLC*: dorsolateral prefrontal cortex; *EC*: entorhinal cortex; *FEF*: frontal eye fields; *GPi*: internal segment of globus pallidus (equivalent to medial pallidum); *HC*: hippocampal cortex; *ITG*: inferior temporal gyrus; *LOF*: lateral orbitofrontal cortex; *MC*: motor cortex; *MDpl*: medialis dorsalis pars paralamellaris; *MDmc*: medialis dorsalis pars magnocellularis; *MDpc*: medialis dorsalis pars parvocellularis; *PPC*: posterior parietal cortex; *PUT*: putamen; *SC*: somatosensory cortex; *SMA*: supplementary motor area; *SNr*: substantia nigra pars reticulata; *STG*: superior temporal gyrus; *VAmc*: ventralis anterior pars magnocellularis; *VApc*: ventralis anterior pars parvocellularis; *VLm*: ventralis lateralis pars medialis; *VLo*: ventralis lateralis pars oralis; *VP*: ventral pallidum; *VS*: ventral striatum; *cdm-*: caudal dorsomedial; *cl-*: caudolateral; *dl-*: dorsolateral; *l-*: lateral; *ldm-*: lateral dorsomedial; *m-*: medial; *mdm-*: medial dorsomedial; *pm-*: posteromedial; *rd-*: rostrodorsal; *rm-*: rostromedial; *vl-*: ventrolateral; *vm-*: ventromedial; *vl-*: ventrolateral.

SNr, and thalamus and ends in one particular cortical area that relates to its function. For example, the *motor* circuit begins in four areas of the frontal cortex related to motor function, projects to the putamen, from there to restricted areas of the globus pallidus or caudolateral SNr, then on to a specific area of the ventrolateral thalamus, and terminates in the supplementary motor area of the cortex. The motor circuit can be divided even more finely into parallel subdivisions serving particular body parts (Alexander, Delong, and Strick 1986; Malach and Graybiel 1986).

All the other circuits so far defined pass through various parts of the caudate, leaving the putamen for the motor circuit only. The other circuits for which there is adequate anatomic and functional evidence include one related to eye movements, two related to cognitive functions, and one to emotional function. One important property of an individual circuit is that lesions at different segments have very similar effects (e.g., Divac, Rosvold, and Szwarcbart 1967; Fuster and Alexander 1973; Alexander, Witt, and Goldman-Rakic 1980).

Other Basal Ganglia Structures   In addition to the cortical input, the striatum has several other important incoming fiber tracts (DiFiglia, Pasik, and Pasik 1978; Carpenter 1986). Two of these fiber tracts originate in basal ganglia structures that may have an important influence on the pathophysiology of HD (figure 5.5A). The *substantia nigra pars compacta* (SNC) and other similar dopaminergic nuclei send many axons to the striatum. This dopaminergic input is thought to have a modulating or "fine tuning" effect on the striatum, but in HD, as the striatal dopamine receptors are gradually lost, the dopamine input becomes relatively excessive.

The *subthalamic nucleus* may also be important in HD pathophysiology. It provides the connection between the lateral and medial pallidum, receiving fibers from the lateral pallidum and sending fibers to the medial pallidum. When the subthalamic nucleus is lesioned, either by stroke in humans (Whittier 1947) or experimentally in primates (Carpenter, Whittier, and Mettler 1950), ballismus results. Ballismus is indistinguishable from severe, high-amplitude chorea (Bruyn and Went 1986). It was given a different name because of its striking severity and its sudden onset following an infarct. It has been suggested that, in HD, striatal pathology may indirectly alter the physiology of the subthalamic nucleus, causing chorea.

The Neurochemistry of the Corpus Striatum

The known and presumed transmitters of the cortical-subcortical circuit are summarized in Figure 5.5B (Graybiel and Ragsdale 1983; Sanberg and Coyle 1984; Calne and Martin 1986). The axons entering the striatum from the cortex are thought to use glutamic acid (GLU) as their transmitter and provide an excitatory stimulus upon the striatal neurons. Most of the spiny output neurons in the neostriatum utilize γ-aminobutyric acid (GABA) as their major transmit-

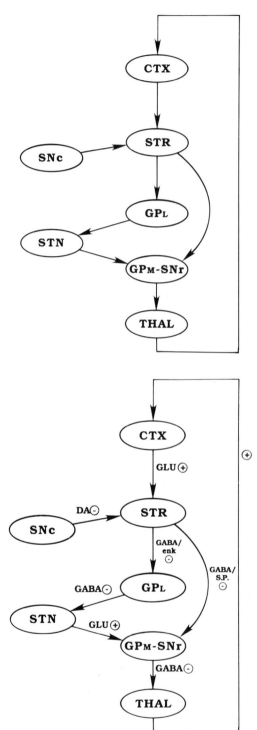

Figure 5.5. (A) Schematic representation of the basal ganglia which demonstrates the maincortical-subcortical circuit as well as two of the subsidiary circuits. *CTX:* cortex; *STR:* striatum; *GPL:* lateral globus pallidus; *GPM-SNr:* medial globus pallidus-substantia nigra reticularis; *THAL:* thalamus; *SNc:* substantia nigra compacta; *STN:* subthalamic nucleus. (B) This figure adds the major neurotransmitters and indicates whether they are excitatory (+) or inhibitory (−). *GLU:* glutamate; *DA:* dopamine; *GABA:* γ-aminobutyric acid; *enk:* enkephalin; *S.P.:* substance P.

ter and inhibit firing in the pallidum. However, in addition to GABA, and in some cases instead of GABA, subpopulations of spiny neurons utilize one or more peptides as transmitters or modulators (Penny, Chang, and Kitai 1986; Penny, Afsharpour, and Kitai 1986; Graybiel 1986). These chemically defined subpopulations of spiny neurons have different target areas in the pallidum with fibers containing met-enkephalin going to lateral pallidum and fibers containing substance P going to medial pallidum (Gerfen 1984).

Most of the aspiny local circuit neurons in the striatum utilize either acetylcholine (aspiny II) or somatostatin (aspiny I). The interneurons synapse both with a variety of axons entering the striatum and with striatal spiny output neurons. Thus the interneurons could provide communication between the parallel inputs from cortex to the striatum and may also modulate the striatal output (DiFiglia 1987), but the extent to which this occurs is still not known.

Pallidal neurons, like the spiny neurons of the striatum, utilize GABA as their transmitter and inhibit the thalamus. Unlike the striatal spiny neurons, however, pallidal neurons do not appear to utilize peptides as transmitters. Thalamic neurons which send their axons to the cortex, closing the circuit, are excitatory to the cortex, but the transmitter has not been identified.

The effect of dopamine input to the striatum from the SNc is complicated, and it may affect different striatal neurons differently. The lateral pallidum (GABAergic) inhibits the subthalamus, which in turn has an excitatory influence (glutamatergic) on the medial pallidum (Kita and Kitai 1987).

Neurochemically Defined Compartments in the Striatum

The striatum was once thought to be relatively homogeneous because its neurons were not layered or otherwise obviously structured as are those in the cerebral cortex. However, when examined with neurochemical markers, the striatum is revealed to be comprised of a series of labyrinths surrounded by a matrix. The labyrinths, also called striosomes or patches because of their cross-sectional appearance, were first noticed as areas of low acetylcholinesterase staining (Graybiel and Ragsdale 1978), but can also be demonstrated by other methods and contain high levels of met-enkephalins. The patches are well defined in the dorsal anterior caudate but gradually become less common toward the putamen. The patches are the site of entry to the striatum for only certain types of fibers, including some from medial limbic cortex and dopamine fibers from the ventral SNc (Gerfen 1984, 1986).

The matrix receives fibers from the motor and sensory cortex and is the exit point for all fibers going to the pallidum-SNr. Both the somatostatinergic (Sandell, Graybiel, and Chesselet 1986) and cholinergic interneurons appear to be limited to the matrix (Graybiel, Baughman, and Eckenstein 1986). The matrix can also be thought of as containing patches or districts. These are defined not neurochemically but by their inputs from restricted cortical areas (e.g., Alexander 1984; Malach and Graybiel 1986).

The concept is beginning to emerge that the dorsal matrix areas of caudate and putamen are related to motor and cognitive functions and that the ventral matrix and patch system is related to limbic or emotion-related input. Because these three functions (motor, cognitive, and emotional) are all disturbed in several basal ganglia diseases, and because the three appear to be related in health, investigators have searched for connections between these two systems. One possibility is that these two systems communicate via the somatostatin interneurons (Gerfen 1984), the dendrites of which enter the patches, and through a variety of indirect pathways (Nauta and Domesick 1981; Nauta 1986; Gerfen, Herkenham, and Thibault 1987; Gerfen, Baimbridge, and Thibault 1987).

In summary, the striatum can be conceived as that segment of the cortical-subcortical circuit which receives input from diverse cortical areas. Inputs from cortical areas serving motor, cognitive, and emotional functions enter in parallel, segregated circuits. Each parallel circuit is modulated by inputs from the substantia nigra compacta and other dopamine nuclei, the subthalamic nucleus, and several other nuclei and emerges as a chemically and anatomically specified pathway (Graybiel 1984). The patch system does not follow this same organizational plan. Its limbic cortical input is modified by dopamine input, but there is no output from the patches to the pallidum.

Because of the convergence in the striatum of fibers from cortical areas serving such diverse functions, injury to this small brain area affects a wide variety of functions and produces the triad of motor, cognitive, and emotional features of HD and other basal ganglia disorders (Folstein and Folstein 1987; McHugh 1987). Just how the parallel matrix circuits interact with each other in the striatum and how the matrix and patch systems may communicate is still under investigation.

Case Example: Obtaining Brains for Research in Huntington's Disease

Mr. Carter was diagnosed with HD the same year as his sister; one year later his daughter became affected. The family was stunned by the realization that three members would become incapacitated and die, and responded by participating in HD research.

Over the course of 10 years Mr. Carter participated in numerous experimental therapeutic trials. He came regularly for examination at the BHDP Research Clinic but refused to take any medication so that he would be eligible to participate "in case a new drug is discovered." Eventually his disease progressed and he required care in a nursing home, where he died 3 years later from aspiration pneumonia after choking on food.

The time of death was 2:00 A.M. The family was promptly notified, and Mrs. Carter was told that the doctor would be in to sign the death certificate the next morning. She had been helped by the BHDP social worker to plan for a "research" autopsy for her husband. She knew, therefore, that the death certificate must accompany the body to Johns Hopkins Hospital and that the body must be transported promptly to the hospital for the brain to be usable in neurochemistry studies. She insisted that the nursing home staff arrange for a physician to sign the death certificate promptly. Next she telephoned a BHDP staff member, who alerted the pathology resident on call and the admissions office to expect a body for autopsy from outside the hospital. The BHDP staff member reviewed the procedures with Mrs. Carter and reminded her to send a telegram to the hospital giving permission for autopsy. The BHDP staff had organized a procedure by which the family member telephones a toll-free number at Western Union and requests that telegram BHDP-9 be sent to Johns Hopkins Hospital. Finally, the family called a previously designated funeral director, who transported the body to Hopkins within two hours of the death.

At autopsy, the brain weighed 950 grams. The brain surface showed moderate atrophy of the frontal and parietal lobes. On cut section, the lateral ventricles were bilaterally and symmetrically enlarged because of atrophy of the caudate and putamen. There was loss of the normal medial caudate convexity into the frontal horn of the lateral ventricles. Additionally, the middle cerebellar peduncles were atrophic bilaterally, as was the basis pontis. Half the brain was frozen for later use in neurochemistry experiments, and the other half was fixed in formalin for diagnostic purposes and neuropathology experiments.

On microscopic examination there was thinning of the cortical ribbon, most evident in the frontal lobes, and possible neuronal loss and glial proliferation of deep layers of both frontal and temporal lobes. Midhippocampal and amygdala sections were unremarkable. Sections of the caudate and putamen showed severe neuronal loss, gliosis, and rarefaction, with some preservation of larger neurons; the anterior putamen was least affected. The globus pallidus also showed mild-to-moderate neuronal loss, gliosis, and marked demyelination, particularly in the lateral pallidum posteriorly. Sections taken from thalamic and subthalamic nuclei were normal. Midbrain sections were remarkable only for mild extracellular neuromelanin. The red nucleus appeared normal. There was neuronal loss in the dentate nucleus of the cerebellum, but the cerebellar hemispheres were normal.

The Corpus Striatum in Huntington's Disease

Gross and Microscopic Neuropathology in HD

The most evident and most constant neuropathologic change in HD is atrophy and neuronal loss in the striatum (figure 5.6). Because patients with advanced disease who come to autopsy have atrophy in many brain areas, this essential neuropathologic change was not clearly noted until 1908 (Jelgersma 1908) and not universally accepted until the 1920s (reviewed by Bruyn 1968). In brains of

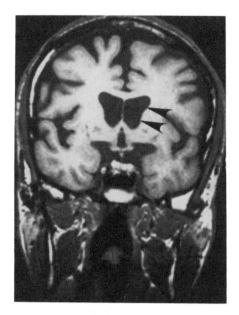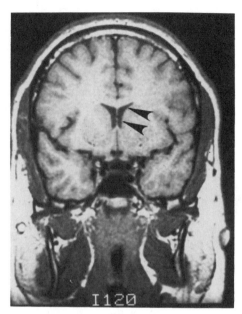

Figure 5.6. Magnetic resonance imaging (MRI) scan of a 31-year-old HD patient (*left*) and an age-matched control subject (*right*). Caudate atrophy can be appreciated by comparing the patient's scan with the control's. The medial border of the right caudate is marked in each figure by arrows.

patients who have died in a cachectic state after many years of illness, atrophy is widespread and loss of brain weight is marked, reduced by as much as 400 grams.

While pathology has been described in many brain areas, the pathology of the components of the cortical-subcortical circuit, particularly the striatum, has been most extensively studied. Many cases and case series have been described in the pathology literature (reviewed by Bruyn 1968). However, only a few studies have attempted to document the amount of atrophy, neuronal loss, and fiber loss by systematic measurement of volume and counting of neurons. In one such morphometric study of six advanced cases, profound loss of neurons was documented in the caudate and putamen (70% reduction) and pallidum (40% reduction). In some brains there was a loss of neurons in the subthalamus (Lange et al. 1976). The axons of the striatal spiny neurons that project to the pallidum (the striatopallidal tract) and the dendrites of pallidal neurons with which they synapse are also severely depleted (Gebbink 1968). Reactive gliosis is usually described in the striatum, and, while the concentration of glial cells is increased because of tissue shrinkage, the absolute numbers of glia are normal to slightly decreased (Lange et al. 1976). The glia appear as they do following a CNS injury, which is why they are described as reactive. A study of the ventrolateral thalamus (the recipient of pallidal output) showed depletion of the small interneurons with sparing of the larger output neurons (Dom, Malfroid, and Baro 1976). Atrophy of the cerebral cortex (the point of origin and termination of the cortical-subcortical circuit) is also commonly observed in HD. Atrophy is particularly evident in frontal and occipital areas, but the type and extent of neuronal changes in cortex have not been agreed upon (Bruyn 1968). An electron microscopic study reported normal cortical neurons (Roos, Bots, and Hermans 1985), but abnormalities in neuronal cytoarchitecture are reported in other studies (e.g., Tellez-Nagel, Johnson, and Terry 1973).

Neuropathologic changes are also evident outside the cortical-subcortical circuit. Cerebellar pathology is commonly described, particularly neuronal loss in the dentate nucleus. Jeste, Barban, and Parisi (1984) demonstrated a 50% reduction in Purkinje cell density in half the brains they examined. Many other parts of the brain have been variously described as atrophic, gliotic, and showing neuronal loss, but cell counts have not been carried out and the changes are not noted in every case, so the significance of these changes is not clear (Bruyn 1968; Roos 1986). Considerable effort has been expended trying to discern neuropathologic differences between choreic HD and the rigid, akinetic Westphal variant commonly seen in juvenile HD, but findings have not been consistent (Roos 1986).

It is clear that while the striatum is most consistently and severely affected, the brains of HD patients who die after many years of illness in a terminal, cachectic state usually have atrophy and neuronal loss in many areas. This widespread neuropathology has been interpreted in two general ways, which are not mutually exclusive. Some pathologists have reasoned that HD must be a multifocal degeneration in which the striatum is the most vulnerable of many vulnerable brain nuclei (e.g., Lange et al. 1976). This view is consistent with the hypothesis (see below) that HD results from a neurotransmitter or receptor defect, which could be present in several brain areas but to which neuronal populations vary in their vulnerability (Robinson and Coyle 1987; Schwarcz and Kohler 1983).

Others have reasoned that the striatum is the site of the essential neuropathologic change, and that other brain areas are injured secondarily as a result of anterograde and retrograde degeneration. This view is supported by a study by Vonsattel et al. (1985), who systematically studied a series of brains chosen to vary as widely as possible in the severity of pathology. An orderly progression of striatal neuropathologic change was discerned, and a scheme for grading the severity of neuropathology in HD was devised (table 5.1). In brains of patients who died early in the disease (although with obvious clinical manifestations), no striatal atrophy or neuronal loss was evident (designated as pathology grade 0). Brains designated as grade I had no grossly visible atrophy, but examiners could appreciate mild neuronal loss, which was limited to the medial, dorsal caudate near the ventricles. However, cell counts revealed that

Table 5.1. Atrophy (A) and Neuronal Depletion (ND) in Huntington's Disease Progress Medial to Lateral

Atrophy Grade	Medial Caudate		Lateral Caudate		Putamen		Lateral Pallidum		Medial Pallidum		Nucleus Accumbens	
	A	ND	A	ND	A	ND	A	ND	A	ND	A	ND
0	0	0	0	0	0	0	0	0	0	0	0	0
I	0	1–2	0	0–1	0	0	0	0	0	0	0	0
II	1	2	1	1	1	1–2	0	0	0	0	0	0
III	2–3	3	2–3	2	2	2–3	1	1	1	0–1	0–1	0–1
IV	4	4	4	4	3	4	2	1–2	2	1–2	1	0–1

Source: Modified from Vonsattel et al. 1985, with permission.

Note: A systematic examination of a series of HD brains chosen for variability in the overall severity of neuropathologic findings (grades 0 to IV) demonstrated that atrophy (A) and neuronal degeneration (ND) begin in the medial caudate and proceed laterally to the putamen and then to the pallidum. Ventral areas (for example, the nucleus accumbens) are normal except in grade III and IV brains.

half the neurons in the caudate had been lost in the grade I brains. In grade II brains there was mild visible atrophy, and neuronal loss had proceeded laterally and ventrally in the caudate and involved the putamen. Grade III and IV brains had progressively more atrophy and neuronal loss amounting to 80% and 95%, respectively.

Neuronal loss proceeds from medial (near the ventricles) to lateral and from dorsal to ventral, as confirmed by cell counts in the caudate (Vonsattell et al. 1985) and putamen (Roos et al. 1985). Except in the most advanced cases, atrophy and neuronal loss in the caudate exceeded that of the putamen, and atrophy and neuronal loss in the striatum exceeded that of the pallidum in all cases. Only in advanced cases was mild atrophy and neuronal loss seen in the pallidum-SNr. Other brain areas were not examined in this series.

While this orderly progression of atrophy and neuronal loss is the general rule, individual brains from patients with typical symptoms during life and from known HD families can be quite varied (Bruyn 1968). Atrophy of the putamen can occur first (Carrosco and Mukherji 1986); some patients with advanced clinical disease, from families documented to have a mutation at the usual chromosome 4 locus, have extremely mild neostriatal findings (Zweig et al. in press); brainstem nuclei and areas of the spinal cord can be prominently affected (Bruyn 1968; reviewed by Zweig et al. in press).

Patterns of Pathology in Striatal Neuronal Populations

Patterns of neuronal loss have been considered in detail in the neostriatum. The spiny neurons and their axons that project to the pallidum are severely depleted. The somatostatin-using aspiny interneurons are relatively spared (Ferrante et al. 1987). It had been thought that the cholinergic interneurons were lost, based on declines in acetylcholinesterase, but new evidence suggests they may be spared (Feigenbaum et al. 1986). Fibers coming into the striatum from other parts of the brain are normal. Striatal glial cells are also somewhat decreased in number but, because of tissue shrinkage, appear to be relatively increased.

In an elegant study, Graveland, Williams, and DiFiglia (1985b) presented evidence that spiny output neurons in the HD striatum may attempt to regenerate. In lateral striatal areas where the neurons were relatively preserved, long, curving dendrites were observed on spiny neurons. These dendrites were longer than average and appeared to follow a curving path, as if searching unsuccessfully for an opportunity to make synaptic contact. In medial striatal areas where only rare spiny neurons remained, these regenerative changes were less often seen and the remaining neurons appeared in the process of degeneration. In addition to providing evidence that neurons may regenerate, the study confirmed that neuronal loss proceeds from medial to lateral in the striatum, as also found by Vonsattel et al. (1985).

The patch-matrix pattern is largely preserved in brains graded 0–II but gradually fades and becomes distorted in brains graded III and IV (Feigenbaum et al. 1986).

Neurotransmitter and Receptor Pathology

Knowledge about the neurochemical changes in HD is limited to the striatum and its direct connections. In general, the findings that have been consistently replicated are indeed consistent with expectations based on neuropathology. The findings are summarized in figure 5.7A.

Transmitter and Receptor Changes Resulting from Neuronal Loss in the Striatum
All the neurotransmitters utilized by the spiny output neurons and the cholinergic aspiny interneurons are gradually depleted in HD. GABA, the most abundant neurotransmitter utilized by the striatal output neurons, is depleted in the striatum and in the pallidum/SNr, to which the spiny neurons project (Perry et al. 1973). The neuropeptides present in striatal output neurons either alone or in combination with GABA (e.g., met-enkephalin, substance P) are also gradually diminished in striatum and pallidum (Ferrante et al. 1986; Feigenbaum et al. 1986; DeSouza et al. 1988). Acetylcholine, the transmitter of aspiny I interneurons, is depleted. Somatostatin, the transmitter on the preserved aspiny II neurons, is increased.

Receptors present on striatal neurons are gradually depleted. These include the glutamate receptors (London et al. 1981), the GABA receptors, the cholinergic receptors, and the dopamine receptors (Reisine et al. 1977; Enna et al. 1976; Whitehouse et al. 1985). GABA receptors are depleted very early in the illness (Walker et al. 1984), supporting the clinical and anatomical evidence that the spiny neuron is dysfunctional long before atrophy can be seen in routine

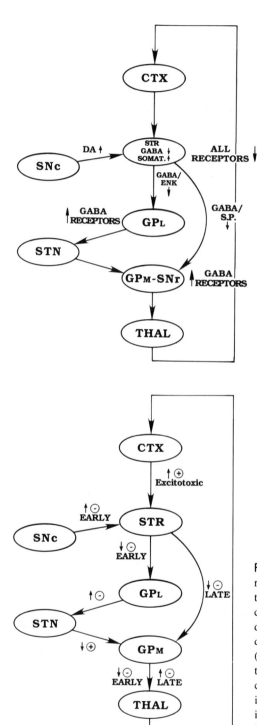

Figure 5.7 (*A*) The major neurotransmitter and receptor changes that have been documented to occur in Huntington's disease. ↑ indicates an increase; ↓ indicates a decrease. *SOMAT:* somatostatin. (*B*) Possible changes in firing patterns that are hypothesized to occur in early and late HD. ↑ ⊕ indicates an increase in excitatory input; ↓ ⊖ indicates a decrease in inhibitory input, etc.

CT scans and before neuronal loss can be appreciated in microscopic sections of striatum.

GABA receptors in the pallidum-SNr neurons are increased in HD brains, as are benzodiazepine receptors which form part of the GABA receptor (Young et al. 1984). These receptors are probably up-regulated in response to decreasing striatal input (Penney and Young 1982; Whitehouse et al. 1985).

Transmitter Changes Reflecting Striatal Inputs Dopamine, contained in incoming fibers from the SNc and other nearby dopaminergic neuronal populations, is either absolutely or relatively increased in the HD striatum. Dopamine release may be up-regulated in response to the decreasing number of dopamine receptors on the striatal neurons.

Receptor and transmitter studies involving structures outside the striatum, pallidum, and substantia nigra have been less systematic, but in general, abnormalities have not been found in the cortex or other brain areas that are variably atrophic. In the cortex, neurotransmitters and receptors have been either normal (DeSouza et al. 1988) or increased (Whitehouse et al. 1985).

Speculations on Clinical-Pathologic Relationships

The Neurochemical Circuitry of the Striatum and the Results of Its Interruption

It is possible to construct a preliminary "wiring diagram" of the cortical-subcortical circuit and some of its subsidiary circuits (figure 5.5B). If HD is presumed to be an illness where nature performs a slowly progressive ablation of the striatal segment of the circuit, the firing changes that are predicted to result from that ablation may be consistent with the clinical findings in HD (Penney and Young 1986).

Symptoms Related to the Major Corticosubcortical Circuit There is some evidence that the spiny neurons, whose axons contain GABA/met-enkephalin and project to the *lateral* pallidum, degenerate earlier in the illness than do the GABA-substance P neurons, which project to the *medial* pallidum. If this is so (figure 5.7B), a unified hypothesis can be made about the early predominance of chorea and the late-appearing parkinsonian-like clinical picture in HD. Under this hypothesis, an early decrease in GABA/enkephalin input to lateral pallidum would result in the disinhibition of the lateral pallidum and the consequent inhibition, or physiological ablation, of the subthalamic nucleus. Ablation of the subthalamic nucleus is known to cause chorea, the predominant motor sign in early HD (Carpenter, Whittier, and Mettler 1950). Experimental ablation of the subthalamic nucleus has been shown to result in decreased firing rates in the medial pallidum (Hamada and DeLong 1988).

Under this same hypothesis, the GABA/substance P neurons which project directly to medial pallidum are gradually lost later in HD. This loss of inhibition on the medial pallidum would gradually lead to a reversal of the earlier balance, with increased firing of the medial pallidum. This is the same firing pattern seen in experimental parkinsonism (DeLong, personal communication).

The net effect both early and late in the illness is to disrupt the functioning of the cortical-subcortical circuit. Reasoning from known functions of the motor circuit (Alexander, DeLong, and Strick 1986), one could expect its disruption to result in a gradually decreasing ability to perform quickly, change sets, and initiate activities. The circuits related to eye movements and cognitive functions probably serve analogous functions and are consistent with the motor, eye movement, and cognitive abnormalities seen in HD.

Symptoms Related to a Loss of Dopaminergic Inhibition   The effect of input from the substantia nigra compacta (SNc) is also changed in HD. Dopaminergic input from the SNc is probably up-regulated in HD in response to declining striatal dopamine receptors. Early in the disease, while some striatal neurons are still functional and react to the excessive dopamine, the balance between dopamine and other striatal neurochemical systems is upset. Some signs and symptoms (particularly chorea and irritability) can be ameliorated early in the disease by dopamine antagonists such as the phenothiazines. Decreasing the available dopamine is thought to restore the balance of neurochemical activity between the substantia nigra and the striatum. However, as the disease progresses, dopamine receptors in the striatum are lost altogether and dopamine antagonists are less useful in controlling involuntary movements. Thus, Penney and Young (1986) suggested that the influence of the dopamine input is lost, resulting in a clinical picture similar to parkinsonism, but due to dopamine receptor loss in the striatum rather than neuronal loss in the substantia nigra.

Symptoms Related to a Disruption of Limbic Input   Reasoning from cortical-subcortical circuit wiring diagrams is plausible when considering the motor and cognitive symptoms in HD, which become progressively worse with time. However, emotional symptoms, particularly depression, can appear quite early in the disorder, sometimes years before the onset of motor and cognitive signs and symptoms. It seems reasonable, therefore, to argue that depression, and possibly other emotional symptoms such as anxiety and irritability, must be related to some function of the dorsal medial caudate, the site of the earliest neuropathologic change (Vonsattel et al. 1985). The patch system is particularly prominent and well defined in this area of the caudate and is the site of cortical limbic input to the striatum. Therefore, I hypothesized that the dorsal medial caudate patches are, among numerous limbic connections to the striatum (Nauta 1986), the site responsible for the early occurrence of mood instability in HD (Folstein and Folstein 1987).

Hypotheses about the Neural Mechanism of Gene Action

While neuroscientists have made many discoveries about the normal function of the striatum and the ways it is changed in HD, at this writing we still do not know how the gene acts to kill the striatal neurons. However, strong hypotheses are emerging.

The Excitotoxin Hypothesis

The best-developed hypothesis is the excitotoxin hypothesis (Coyle and Schwarcz 1976; McGeer and McGeer 1976). The concept that excitatory brain chemicals (especially glutamate and its structural analogues) could be toxic to neurons originated with Lucas and Newhouse (1957), who observed that when monosodium glutamate was injected into the retina, neurons degenerated. Olney (1969) reported similar neuronal degeneration in the brain and noted that fibers passing through or terminating in the injected area were spared. Coyle and Schwarcz (1976) injected kainic acid, a glutamate structural analog, into the striatum of rats and were able to approximate the striatal neuropathology of HD, which is characterized by a loss of striatal neurons and sparing of fibers entering the striatum. Similar effects are obtained with other glutamate analogues, quinolinate, N-methyl-D-aspartate (NMDA), and quisqualate. All these compounds bind to glutamate receptors which transmit excitatory neural impulses. Currently, at least three types of glutamate receptors have been defined based on the glutamate analogues for which they have the highest affinity. The best characterized is the NMDA receptor, which is also activated by quinolinate. The other two are selectively activated by kainate and quisqualate, respectively. Only the NMDA receptor contains a transmitter-activated calcium channel (Cotman et al. 1987).

The finding that glutamate analogues could mimic the neuropathology of HD led to the hypothesis that the HD gene alters the glutamate transmitter system. Glutamate is the most common excitatory neurotransmitter, and abundant glutamate-containing fibers enter the striatum from the cortex (Schwarcz et al. 1981). Several possible types of abnormality of the glutamate system are possible. There may be excessive release of glutamate or related excitatory neurotransmitters, a failure of the re-uptake system, an increased sensitivity of the glutamate receptors to glutamate, or a variety of abnormalities of other aspects of the glutamate receptor. Alternatively, post-synaptic mechanisms (within the neuronal cell body) could be defective (Choi 1988). Currently, these hypotheses are still speculative, and the damage produced by the excitatory transmission system could be a second order effect of a yet undiscovered neurophysiologic mechanism.

The most direct evidence for involvement of the NMDA receptor in the pathogenesis of HD has been provided by the finding of dramatic loss of NMDA receptors in the HD putamen (Young et al. 1988). This loss was out of proportion to the loss of other types of receptors in the striatum, including GABA, benzodiazepine, muscarinic, cholinergic, and quisqualate. In another study, Cross, Slater, and Reynolds (1986) reported reduced numbers of glutamate uptake sites in the terminals of corticostriate fibers in HD patients.

Recent evidence from experiments in neuron cultures further suggests that the failure of corticostriate fibers to take up glutamate could be one mechanism for excitotoxic damage. When NMDA receptors are excessively stimulated, a sodium/calcium channel remains chronically open, resulting in an excess influx of calcium into the neuron. The elevated intraneuronal calcium activates several processes leading to the formation of excessive free radicals (such as superoxides and peroxides) which are cytotoxic to the neuron (Machlin and Bendick 1987; Choi 1988). Glutamate analogues have similar effects on neurons in culture, causing them to swell and die. The damage can be prevented by pretreatment of the neurons with anti-oxidants such as α-tocopherol and idebenone (Miyamoto et al. 1988). When rats were given intraperitoneal injections of these antioxidants, followed by glutamate analogue injections to the striatum, the behavioral effects of striatal glutamate toxicity were markedly attenuated (Miyamoto et al., submitted).

There is some evidence that neuronal degeneration in HD may result from oxidative stress and free radical formation. May and Gray (1985) reported that cultured fibroblasts from HD patients are particularly vulnerable to peroxidative damage. Moreover, striatal neurons that express the reducing agent NADPH diaphorase are spared in HD. NADPH also prevents glutamate toxicity in a neuronal cell line (DeLong et al. 1988).

The Oxidative Phosphorylation Hypothesis

Independent of the evidence from the excitotoxic hypothesis that oxidative stress may be involved in the pathogenesis of HD, an oxidative stress hypothesis has been suggested based on observation of the paternal transmission effect. The finding that the symptoms of HD begin at a younger age when the gene has been transmitted by the father than when it has been transmitted by the mother (Merritt et al. 1969) suggested the possibility that the age at onset might be controlled by mitochondrial genes (Myers et al. 1983). Nearly all mitochondria are contributed to the fetus in the cytoplasm of the maternal ovum; very few are found in sperm with its minimal amount of cytoplasm. Mitochondrial genes are entirely devoted to the manufacture of enzymes used in oxidative phosphorylation (the cytochrome oxidase cascade). The mitochondria also take up intracellular calcium. These enzymes vary somewhat from one person to the next, apparently resulting in a variation in the efficiency with which oxygen molecules are transformed to water. Thus, the concentration of toxic free radicals, such as hydroxyl radicals and hydrogen peroxide, that escape the system also varies from one person to the next (Wallace 1987). This means that persons with more efficient cytochrome oxidase enzymes have a lower concentration of free radicals in their cells, including their neurons.

In the case of a woman who has the HD gene, the age at onset must be sufficiently late if she is to bear children. Such a person would be hypothesized to have an "efficient" oxidative phosphorylation system and would transmit the same mitochondrial-dependent system to all her children, including those who also inherited the HD gene. Men with HD who became fathers would be similarly selected for having an efficient mitochondrial oxidative phosphorylation system, but the mitochondrial system transmitted to their children is contributed by the unaffected mother, who has encountered no such selective pressure. Therefore, the mitochondrial oxidative phosphorylation enzymes inherited by the offspring of affected fathers will reflect the general population frequencies of the various enzyme types.

One toxic result of the excessive stimulation of glutamate receptors is the generation of an excessive number of free radicals inside neurons. Persons with the HD gene coupled with an efficient mitochondrial phosphorylation system would, under this hypothesis, tend to have a late onset because free radicals would be inactivated more efficiently, slowing the rate of neuronal death. Conversely, the HD gene coupled with a relatively inefficient oxidative phosphorylation system would inactivate free radicals poorly, so onset would be hastened.

Summary and Conclusions

HD is predominantly a disease of the striatum and the recipient of its output, the pallidum. The neuropathology is characterized by atrophy and neuronal loss that usually begins in the medial caudate, near the ventricles, and progresses laterally and ventrally. The brains of patients who have lived for many years with HD show widespread atrophy, but neurochemical abnormalities are most striking in the striatum.

The striatum receives its primary input from cortical areas serving motor, cognitive, and emotional functions, and it serves to modulate and chemically specify a wide variety of information. It is postulated that damage to the striatum can account for the motor, cognitive, and emotional disturbances in HD. It is also postulated that the HD gene exerts its effect by influencing the excitatory glutamate corticostriate pathway so the striatal neurons are excessively stimulated and gradually destroyed by excessive free radical concentrations, which are a direct outcome of excitotoxicity.

6

Epidemiology

The disease . . . exists, so far as I know, almost exclusively on
the east end of Long Island.
—HUNTINGTON, 1872

The frequency of Huntington's disease in the population is usually expressed in terms of prevalence or incidence. Prevalence is the proportion of a
surveyed population having an illness at a particular time and is usually expressed as cases per 100,000 population. Prevalence estimates are frequently
used to assess the burden of the illness on society and to estimate service needs
(Lilienfeld and Lilienfeld 1980). Incidence is the number of new cases that
appear during a specified time period and can be estimated from prevalence or
can be measured directly. The success of interventions directed toward treatment or prevention can be assessed by comparing the actual incidence with
what would have been expected if an intervention had not been undertaken.

Community surveys of HD are also a useful means of finding patients and
their families, many of whom are undiagnosed and unknown to any community
source of care. If methods for treating or preventing HD were available, large-
scale community surveys of HD would be needed to inform HD families that
such options were available.

A survey of HD can also be used to gain an appreciation of the range of
clinical features in a sample of HD patients which is unbiased by referral to a
particular agency or source of care. Many of the clinical data presented in
chapters 2, 3, and 4 were based on the systematic examination of such an
unbiased sample.

This chapter discusses some of the difficulties involved in estimating the
prevalence and incidence of HD; it describes the findings of the major population surveys of HD that have been carried out in various parts of the world; and,
finally, it delineates some issues that need to be considered when planning and
implementing a community survey of HD.

Case Example: The Documentation of Affected Members of a Family in the Maryland HD Survey

The Baltimore Huntington's Disease Project (BHDP) carried out a survey of HD in Maryland to estimate the prevalence of HD on the last U.S. Decennial Census Day, 1 April 1980. One of the methods used to find HD patients living in Maryland was to contact and examine all patients given a discharge diagnosis of HD by any general hospital in the state. The survey staff obtained permission to call the family (figure 6.1) of one of these patients, Marilyn Daniels. As the proband, she is indicated on the pedigree drawing by an arrow and as person 4.14, the fourteenth individual in the fourth generation. Mrs. Daniels had been hospitalized for anemia but had told her physician that she also had Huntington's disease. This was listed as a secondary diagnosis on the discharge summary and was entered into the computerized diagnosis file of the hospital. Her name was also provided to the survey staff by the neurologist who had made the diagnosis earlier. In the course of exploring the family history with the patient's mother, we discovered that Mrs. Daniels's brother, James (4.13), had suffered several falls over the past few years, had become irritable, and had lost his job. He was examined and found to be affected with HD. He told the survey staff that he had a child (5.8) born out of wedlock, and he agreed to contact the child's mother to inform her of the child's risk for HD. At the time of his call to the child's mother, the child was being evaluated for school failure and short stature and had been diagnosed as having growth failure of unknown etiology. She was examined by the BHDP Research Clinic survey staff and diagnosed as having juvenile HD.

Two of Mrs. Daniels's affected cousins (4.9, 4.10) were not located during the survey and were, therefore, not counted in the prevalence estimate. They were the identical twin sons of a family member who had died during World War II before the onset of symptoms of HD. The twins had been reared by their mother, who knew nothing about the father's family or his risk for HD. One twin was thought to have a movement disorder secondary to chronic alcoholism but, when the other twin developed the same symptoms, the treating physician entertained the diagnosis of hereditary chorea and referred both twins to the BHDP Research Clinic at Johns Hopkins. Genealogic investigation revealed their relationship to Mrs. Daniels's family.

In summary, at the time of the statewide HD survey, only one member of the family, Mrs. Daniels, had been officially diagnosed and could be found through the sources of medical care being used in the survey. Through exploration of the family history, the survey staff discovered two more family members who had the disease. One of these (5.8) had been given another diagnosis, and the other (4.13) had not yet been seen by any of the sources of care being used by the survey to locate cases. Two other affected relatives (4.9 and 4.10) were unknown to any of the family members and also unknown to any source of care.

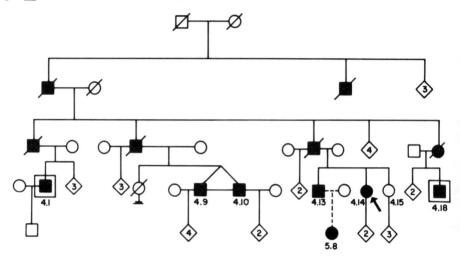

○ □ PRESENTLY UNAFFECTED
● ■ ALIVE AND AFFECTED ON PREVALENCE DAY, 4-1-80
◉ ▣ BECAME SYMPTOMATIC AFTER 4-1-80

Figure 6.1. The proband in this family (4.14, designated by an arrow) was ascertained in the Maryland HD survey by two sources, a general hospital diagnosis and her neurologist. Two other affected family members (4.13 and 5.8) were found only through information given by the family. Two additional members (4.9 and 4.10) were affected on prevalence day, but had not yet been diagnosed and were also unknown to the family members from whom the survey staff were gathering information. Therefore, they were not counted in the prevalence estimate. Individuals 4.1 and 4.18 became symptomatic after prevalence day.

Therefore, although they were living in Maryland and affected with HD on 1 April 1980, the day on which prevalence was estimated, they were not included in the prevalence estimate.

Two additional family members (4.1 and 4.18) are known by the BHDP Research Clinic to have become symptomatic after prevalence day.

Methods Used to Estimate the Prevalence of Huntington's Disease

The prevalence of a disorder is defined as the number of people who are alive and symptomatic during a specified time period, divided by the population at risk for the condition. Epidemiologists use *at risk* to designate the population in which the condition under study is likely to occur, rather than that portion of the population at some specific genetic risk. Each aspect of the definition of prevalence has inherent uncertainties, so prevalence is always an estimate. The estimate will depend on whether patients are required to be alive and symptomatic on one specific day or whether some longer period of time is used, on the age distribution and ethnic mix of the population, on the diagnostic criteria required for inclusion as a case, and on the effectiveness of the methods that have been used to find the cases.

Most of the large HD surveys have estimated *point prevalence*: the number of patients living and symptomatic on a given day, usually a national census day when an accurate estimate of the total population of the area surveyed is available. Most of the surveys have been undertaken in populations of western European origin, the population thought to be at highest risk for HD. They have included the whole population in the denominator, thus estimating *simple point prevalence*. The actual prevalence is higher than the simple estimate for the population between the ages of 30 and 70 years (the age range of most of the symptomatic cases), and actual prevalence is very low in children and in the elderly, ages at which HD is rarely seen.

The number of individuals found in the survey who are counted as having HD also depends on the *diagnostic criteria* used for HD. Because patients with HD can present in such a variety of ways, any set of criteria will exclude some cases. For example, if motor symptoms are required, patients who have only cognitive or emotional abnormalities will not be counted. If a positive family history is required, a few cases will have to be omitted because affected relatives cannot be documented. Surveys have made different decisions about diagnostic criteria depending on the primary purpose of the survey, as discussed below. Finally, prevalence estimates are powerfully influenced by the effectiveness of the *methods of case ascertainment*. In general, the more thorough the search, the greater the proportion of patients found. The proportion of cases missed will depend on how well informed the investigators were about where HD patients would be expected to be registered, the number of HD patients who are registered under another diagnosis, cooperation of agencies in reporting cases, accessibility of records, willingness of families to participate, thoroughness with which reported families are investigated for other affected members, and, finally, proportion of symptomatic cases registered with one of the agencies used in ascertainment.

While it is clear that many cases are missed because of incomplete ascertainment, it has been difficult to devise ways of estimating the number missed. Methods have been constructed that utilize the proportion of cases ascertained through multiple sources as a means of estimating the number of cases that were not ascertained by any source (Wittes, Colton, and Sidel 1974). This method requires that methods of ascertainment be independent from one another (i.e., being registered with one source does not make it more likely that the same case is also registered with another source). The method also requires that cases be ascertained independently from each other (i.e., finding one case is not dependent upon having found another case). This second requirement is not met for dominantly inherited disorders, because the ascertainment of one individual in the family frequently results in a subsequent ascertainment of one or more of the patient's affected family members.

Estimates of Prevalence

Estimates Derived from Populations of Western European Origin

Estimates of Simple Point Prevalence   Many surveys of HD have been carried out during this century in populations of predominantly western European origin, in whom HD is most prevalent. Six of these can be readily compared with each other: the surveys in Michigan (Reed et al. 1958; Reed and Neel 1959), western Scotland (Bolt 1970), Queensland, Australia (Wallace 1972), Sweden (Mattsson 1974a, 1974b), the Gwent and Glamorgan districts of Wales (Walker et al. 1981), and Maryland (Folstein et al. 1986, 1987). All of these surveys used multiple sources of case ascertainment, included genealogical investigations of each proband, surveyed populations living in geographically defined areas, and employed the point prevalence method. Diagnostic criteria were specified in the surveys of Sweden and Maryland, both requiring motor symptoms for diagnosis. The Michigan and western Scotland patients were said to be medically diagnosed and were examined whenever possible. The text of the Queensland survey implies that diagnosis required a movement disorder. The Welsh study gave no criteria, but the investigators say that motor abnormalities, intellectual deficits, and a positive family history were required (Audrey Tyler, personal communication, 1988). The Swedish, Scottish, Welsh, and Australian surveys included only Caucasians, but the populations of Michigan and Maryland included whites and American blacks, and the prevalence for each race was estimated separately.

Table 6.1 shows that the Caucasian prevalence rates in these four surveys differ by about 90%, ranging from 4.1 to 7.5 cases per 100,000 population. The prevalence reported in the Michigan survey (the earliest modern one), where ascertainment sources were limited to institutions, is probably more of an underestimate than the others. Since the other studies used essentially identical

Table 6.1. Point Prevalence Estimates in Caucasians (per 100,000 People)

Study	Location	Prevalence Day	Prevalence
Reed et al. 1958	Michigan	4/01/40	4.1
Bolt 1970	West Scotland	6/30/60	5.2
Wallace 1972	Queensland, Australia	1/01/69	6.3
Mattsson 1974	Sweden	7/01/65	4.7
Walker et al. 1981	South Wales	4/ /71	7.5
Folstein et al. 1987	Maryland	4/01/80	5.3

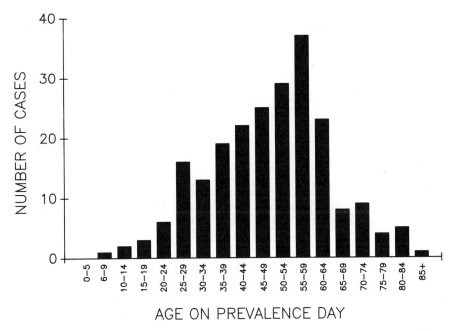

Figure 6.2. The age of the HD patients who were affected and living in Maryland on 1 April 1980, varied from 8 to 91, but most were between the ages of 40 and 59. Thus, although the simple prevalence on that day was 5.3 per 100,000 people, the prevalence of HD in the 40 to 59 age group was 12.5 per 100,000. (See also table 6.2.)

methods, it must be presumed that the prevalence of HD varies somewhat within populations of western European origin, possibly depending on the initial gene frequency in the population and on how isolated the population has remained in succeeding years. The most reliable estimate of simple point prevalence of HD in Caucasians, therefore, appears to vary between 5 and 7 cases per 100,000 total population.

Among the other surveys of populations of western European origin, prevalence estimates range from 2.2 to 8.4 per 100,000 (Panse 1942; Bickford and Ellison 1953; Brothers and Meadows 1955; Heathfield 1967; Oliver 1970; Heathfield and McKenzie 1971; Wendt and Drohm 1972; Marx 1973; Shokeir 1975a). This variation is not easy to explain from the published documents, but it seems more likely to result from methodological differences of the type discussed earlier than from such a wide variation in the actual prevalence of the disorder.

Age-Specific Point Prevalence from the Maryland Survey   From the age distribution of the Maryland population on 1 April 1980, and the age distribution of HD patients in the Maryland survey (figure 6.2), we estimated the age-specific

Table 6.2. Age-Specific Prevalence of Huntington's Disease in the
Maryland Survey (per 100,000 People)

Age Groups	N	Age-Specific Prevalence
(0–19)	6	0.5
(20–39)	54	3.8
(40–59)	113	12.5
(60+)	50	8.7
Overall prevalence	223	5.3

prevalence of HD in Maryland on 1 April 1980 (table 6.2). The prevalence
varied from 0.5 per 100,000 for ages 0 to 19 years to 12.5 per 100,000 for ages
40 to 59. This means that HD is more common in the adult population than is
implied by the simple point prevalence estimates. The number of symptomatic
cases also varies with the age distribution of the population. HD heterozygotes
born during the postwar "baby boom" of 1946–1959 are currently becoming
symptomatic, so that in the United States there are more HD patients, and thus
more requests for services than ever before.

The Prevalence of HD in Some Isolated European Populations

There are a few isolated populations of western European origin in which the
prevalence of HD is unusually high (table 6.3). In most cases, the high prevalence appears to have resulted from a founder effect. When a gene is introduced
into a population—either by mutation or by immigration into the community of
a person with the gene—and when persons with that gene reproduce at a rate
that is even slightly higher than that of the community, the disease or trait will
increase in prevalence in that community. The occurrence of an immigrating
founder has been documented in Tasmania (Brothers 1949, 1964), the island of
Mauritius off the South African coast (Hayden 1979), and around Lake Maracaibo in Venezuela (Avila-Giron 1973). Other areas that have claimed to have
an unusually high prevalence are the Moray Firth in Scotland (Lyon 1962) and

Table 6.3. Isolated Populations with a High Prevalence of Huntington's
Disease Attributed to the Immigration of an Affected Individual

Study	Location	Prevalence per 100,000
Brothers 1949	Tasmania	17.4
Avila-Giron 1973	Lake Maracaibo, Venezuela	700
Hayden 1979	Mauritius	46

an isolated region of northern Sweden (Sjogren 1936). These latter claims are based on small numbers of patients living in small populations, so the estimates are likely to be unstable.

Isolated populations with a high prevalence of HD have been valuable for genetic linkage studies because scientists could be virtually certain that all members of one extended kindred would share the same mutation for Huntington's disease. The study of the Venezuelan population around Lake Maracaibo led to the discovery of the approximate location of the HD gene (Gusella et al. 1983). The story of this discovery is related in more detail in the next chapter.

The Prevalence of HD in Other Ethnic Groups

Reports of individuals and families with HD have come from many countries (Bruyn 1968), but prevalence estimates in populations other than western European have been limited to American blacks (considered a mixed-race population), South African mixed-race blacks, native South Africans, and Japanese. For the most part, these surveys have necessarily been less systematic than those previously described, because of the apparent rarity of the condition and, in some cases, because of social and cultural circumstances within the populations surveyed.

American Blacks   HD has been reported in American blacks since 1890, only 18 years after Huntington's original paper (reviewed by Folstein et al. 1987). Three blacks with HD were found in the Michigan survey, and the investigators refer to two or three other black patients who could not be documented adequately. The estimated prevalence rate within the Michigan black population, based on the three well-documented cases (table 6.4), was only 1.5 per 100,000 blacks in Michigan. However, the authors estimated that the three cases count-

Table 6.4. Prevalence of Huntington's Disease in Blacks and Whites

Study	Location	Prevalence Day	Prevalence		
			Total	White	Black
Reed et al. 1958	Michigan	4/1/40	4.12	4.23[a]	1.44[b]
Wright et al. 1981	South Carolina	—	—	4.8	0.97[b]
Hayden 1981	South Africa	—	—	2.22	2.11[b]
					0.01[c]
Folstein et al. 1987	Maryland	4/1/80	5.15	5.94	6.37[b]

[a]Estimated from data.
[b]Mixed-race blacks (American blacks have been estimated to have 1/3 "Caucasian-origin" genes, on average (Neel and Schull 1954)).
[c]native Africans, without known admixture with Caucasians.

ed were not statistically different from the number expected (8.3 cases) if the frequency of HD in blacks was equal to that in whites.

A survey focused on American blacks (Still 1977; Wright, Still, and Abramson 1981) was reported from South Carolina. Based on a limited investigation, the investigators estimated the prevalence in blacks at only 0.97 cases per 100,000 population. This estimate was based on 9 patients living on January 1980 in the South Carolina black population of approximately 900,000.

In the Maryland survey (1980–1983), 61 blacks with HD were found. This represents a point prevalence of HD of 6.37 per 100,000 blacks living in Maryland on 1 April 1980, an unexpectedly high figure and not significantly different from the prevalence in whites in the same survey. Even if 29 cases contributed by one large family are excluded, the prevalence is still higher than any previously reported in blacks. The diagnosis was confirmed neuropathologically in at least one family member from 6 of the 20 kindreds (including the large one). In two black families, the disease was linked to the HD locus on chromosome 4 (Folstein, Phillips et al. 1985; Zweig et al. in press). The high prevalence found in Maryland blacks was, therefore, not likely a consequence of misdiagnosis.

There are two possible reasons for the high prevalence of HD in Maryland blacks. First, the prevalence could be increasing in blacks. Black reproductive rates are high, so once the gene was introduced into the black population, the number of cases would be expected to increase at a faster rate than in the white population. However, the prevalence was calculated using the black population as the denominator, which suggests that HD is increasing at a faster rate than the black population as a whole.

The second possible reason for the high prevalence is that previous surveys have underestimated the prevalence in blacks because of misdiagnosis and failure to find known cases. The BHDP survey of Maryland documented significantly more misdiagnosis in blacks than in whites (Folstein et al. 1987). There appeared to be several possible reasons for misdiagnosis. First, HD is not expected in blacks and was, therefore, not often considered in the differential diagnosis of a neurodegenerative disease. Second, genealogies are frequently hard to obtain, so the diagnosis of HD could not always be documented when it was entertained. Third, clinical presentation in blacks is somewhat different from that in whites (as discussed in chapter 8), making diagnosis more difficult.

Even blacks known to have HD were often not found through the usual sources of ascertainment (Folstein et al. 1987). Many black patients were found only through the state Department of Social Services, a source of ascertainment that other surveys have not used. Meticulous genealogical explorations of families of ascertained cases turned up 17 affected individuals who were not reported by any other source. Cases were also found by searching the surname index at the state psychiatric hospital that had served blacks exclusively until 1962.

In most cases, it was not possible to document a Caucasian origin of the HD gene in the black families. The largest black kindred was traced back to 1852, without finding any white ancestors. An affected white ancestor could be documented for only 1 of the 23 black kindreds but, because genealogical documentation of blacks is scant, more cases may have been due to racial admixture. Some of the black families found in the Maryland survey are related to the kindreds reported from South Carolina.

In summary, it appears that HD may be more common in American blacks than was previously thought. If this is the case, it may not be possible to account for all the black cases by postulating that HD is a recent introduction into the American black population by racial admixture with whites. If the prevalence is confirmed to be equal to that in whites, it is possible that, in addition to racial admixture, an HD mutation may have been brought from Africa.

Native South Africans and Mixed-Race Blacks   HD has been reported in African blacks since 1935. (For review, see Wright, Still, and Abramson 1981.) Hayden systematically surveyed the South African population in 1979 and found 11 African patients with HD for whom there was no evidence of racial admixture or any known exposure to the white population (Hayden and Beighton 1977). These cases gave an estimated prevalence of only 0.6 cases per million population. Because of social conditions, Hayden's access to cases was limited, and the estimated prevalence may be even more of an underestimate than is usual for HD. But it can be safely concluded that, although HD is rare in Africans, it definitely exists.

During the same survey, Hayden (1981) found, as did the Maryland survey, that prevalences in white and mixed-race black South Africans were almost the same—2.2 and 2.1 per 100,000 population, respectively—although he found a much lower prevalence in both groups than is usual in surveys of Western populations.

Japan   Japan is the only Asian country in which HD has been systematically surveyed. The first Japanese case was reported in 1927, apparently without a family history but with the diagnosis confirmed pathologically. Since that time, cases and families have been reported throughout Japan, but the prevalence is quite low. The one systematic survey of a Japanese prefecture estimated the prevalence at 4.5 per million, about 10% of the usually quoted prevalence in Western countries (Narabayashi 1973). All indications are that the disease, despite its rarity, is the same condition seen in the West. The same clinical syndrome and neuropathologic findings are reported.

Estimating the Incidence of Huntington's Disease

There are several ways to estimate the incidence of HD, the number of new cases per year in the population. The simplest method is to divide the prevalence by the average duration of the illness from onset to death. In a population of one million people with a stable prevalence rate of 50 per million, the expected incidence of HD would be 3 new cases per year, assuming an average duration of illness of 16 years.

A second method, utilized by Harper et al. (1979), predicts incidence rates based on a life-table method that takes into account the number of persons at risk for HD in the population and whether their grandparents or parents are affected, along with their ages and the age-of-onset distribution of the illness. This method requires a complete ascertainment of persons at risk for HD in the population. Such persons are not ordinarily documented by their sources of health care as being at risk for HD. Therefore, they can be found only through their affected family members. This is a difficult task in a highly mobile nation such as the United States, where many persons at risk are living in a different geographical area from their affected family members. This means they can be ascertained only if they know they are at risk and then make themselves known to the survey staff.

In Wales, where the population is relatively stable, complete ascertainment of the at-risk population has been possible. The life-table method results in an incidence estimate of about ten cases per year in south Wales. The method of dividing prevalence by the average duration of illness gives an estimate of eight new cases per year for that population. Thus, the two methods give reasonably similar estimates in this instance.

A third method for estimating incidence is to count the cases that become symptomatic in a given year. This method could be used in populations where there is both national health care and registration of all new cases. But for most countries this method would be hampered by many administrative difficulties and has not been utilized in HD.

Estimating the Number of Persons at Risk for Huntington's Disease

The at-risk population is made up of individuals with the HD gene who have not yet shown symptoms (*asymptomatic heterozygotes*), and the offspring of HD patients who did not inherit the gene (*normal homozygotes*) but whose genotype cannot be determined because they have not yet lived past the age when symptoms might begin.* The number of asymptomatic heterozygotes in a population, relative to the number of symptomatic heterozygotes, can be estimated from data on the prevalence, duration of illness, and average age at onset. On this basis, Reed et al. (1958) estimated that about 40% of heterozygotes were symptomatic at any one time, so all heterozygotes are equal to 2.5 times the number of symptomatic cases ($2.5 \times 40\% = 100\%$). Because there are an equal

---

*This presumes that most or all persons at risk for HD had no access to, or did not choose to have, presympatomatic testing for HD.

number of affected and unaffected offspring, the total number of heterozygotes will equal the number of persons at risk who do not have the gene.

Conneally (1984) suggested that the total at-risk population can be approximated by the following method:

total at-risk population = asymptomatic heterozygotes +
                               homozygotic normal offspring of HD
                               patients

asymptomatic heterozygotes = 2.5 × symptomatic cases − symptomatic
                                  cases

homozygotic normal at-risks = all heterozygotes or
                                = 2.5 × symptomatic cases

Therefore,

total at-risk population = 5 × symptomatic cases − symptomatic
                               cases

Conneally (1984) derived an estimate that is slightly different from that of Reed and Neel because he assumed, based on the National HD Roster's duration-of-illness data, that 33%, rather than 40%, of heterozygotes are symptomatic at any given time.

The Uses of Prevalence and Incidence Estimates

Despite the limitations of our ability to estimate accurately the number of symptomatic patients, asymptomatic heterozygotes, and persons at risk, the available methods can be used for some purposes. If, for instance, the domiciles of patients who were symptomatic on the day of a prevalence estimate were recorded, the need for both out-patient services and chronic care beds in a given catchment area could be estimated and projected. For example, in the Maryland survey 28% of the 217 patients who were symptomatic on prevalence day were institutionalized (unpublished data), suggesting the need for approximately 60 chronic care beds for HD in Maryland.

Estimates of the future prevalence and estimates of the level of need for genetic counseling and presymptomatic testing services could be projected if the survey collects data on the numbers and ages of offspring of the patients in the sample.

Changes in incidence can be used to assess the effectiveness of a planned intervention aimed at the prevention of HD. The Wales survey estimated that the incidence of HD has been fairly constant in Wales since 1900 (Harper et al. 1979). This estimate will form the baseline with which the effectiveness of their genetic counseling program for persons at risk can be measured.

Issues to Be Considered in Planning a Survey of Huntington's Disease

Is a Survey Needed?

A full-scale survey of HD is time consuming and expensive and is not needed to answer some kinds of clinical and laboratory research questions. For example, a successful therapeutic drug trial depends on the selection of cooperative, reliable subjects with supportive families, while studies requiring brain tissue need a source of patients who have advanced disease. On the other hand, if the goal is to plan for service needs, evaluate the effect of a preventive intervention, estimate the size of HD families relative to the population (genetic fitness, see chapter 7), estimate the distribution of age at onset, or document the distribution of particular clinical features in the HD population, then a representative sample is required, and this can be obtained only from a systematic population survey.

A representative survey population is not essential for genetic linkage studies in HD but can be extremely helpful in ascertaining the large families necessary for such work. Genealogic exploration of numerous, independently ascertained survey subjects usually results in finding common ancestors, thus enlarging the kindreds. In the Maryland survey, genealogic investigation of probands often resulted in doubling or tripling the numbers of family members known to be related, so instead of three small uninformative families there was one large, useful one.

Another important purpose of a survey is providing information about HD and about presymptomatic testing to persons at risk. Many at-risk persons are unaware of their risk and, therefore, cannot respond to public announcements of offers to provide information or presymptomatic testing. Many uninformed persons at risk may be reached through affected relatives who would be identified in a survey.

Planning a Survey

Before making decisions about diagnostic criteria, ascertainment sources, or the methods to be used for clinical evaluation of patients found, the investigator must have in mind the questions to be answered by the survey, and an estimate of the human and financial resources available. For example, to estimate mutation rates, a positive family history should not be required as one of the diagnostic criteria. If resources are scarce, sources of ascertainment can be limited to those that will provide the largest number of cases. To investigate the rate of psychiatric disorder, practical and valid methods for its documentation must be developed.

For the most part, decisions about methods of clinical evaluation are particular to the survey. The clinical instruments used in the Maryland survey (included in appendix 1) were designed to answer questions about the prevalence and type of psychiatric disorder associated with HD, the pattern of motor signs at particular stages of illness, and the frequency and severity of dementia. On the other hand, diagnostic criteria, selection of sources of ascertainment, and strategies for gaining access to cases found through those sources are issues common to all surveys and will be discussed here.

Diagnostic Criteria and Methods   Choices and dilemmas concerning diagnostic criteria include whether to include cases with only psychiatric symptoms, whether to require motor symptoms (and if so which ones), and whether to require a positive family history.

It seems reasonable to use psychiatric symptoms to date the onset of the illness (as was done in the Michigan survey) if the prevalence day is several years earlier than the time of the survey. Patients with motor signs at the time of the survey can be retrospectively designated as affected on the prevalence day based on the presence of psychiatric symptoms at that time. In surveys carried out concurrently with prevalence day, it is better to use only motor manifestations to avoid an overinclusion of persons at risk who have psychiatric symptoms for reasons other than HD (Folstein, Franz et al. 1983; Dewhurst, Oliver, and McKnight 1970). We would not suggest using major affective disorder as an indicator of the presence of HD, because some patients have episodes of this syndrome for many years before the onset of HD motor symptoms or dementia associated with a gradually worsening illness.

Even though chorea is the classic (i.e., relating to a class) type of abnormal movement in HD, it is not an adequate diagnostic criterion. As discussed in Chapter 2, patients with HD may have a variety of involuntary and voluntary motor abnormalities, and serious underascertainment would result from the exclusive requirement of chorea for diagnosis. Clinical judgment and experience are required to diagnose HD when chorea is not present, and one can sometimes be certain only when there is a confirming family history.

Estimation of mutation rate requires the inclusion of cases with a negative family history who have typical symptoms, whereas ascertainment of cases for use in most other HD research would exclude such cases. The difficulty is in deciding when the family history is actually negative. A thorough genealogic evaluation of every case reported to have a negative family history requires considerable human resources, cooperation of numerous family members, access to old medical records, and, ideally, paternity testing when no affected family members can be found (Wendt and Drohm 1972). The Maryland survey required either a positive family history or one that was unobtainable by reason of unknown paternity or adoption. Patients for whom no affected family members could be found after a thorough genealogic evaluation were included as affected with HD only if the diagnosis was confirmed by autopsy.

All these suggestions for diagnostic criteria require that each person reported as having HD be examined by a clinician experienced with HD, or have medical records which clearly document the symptoms and course, along with a positive family history. Numerous cases mistaken for HD will be reported to the survey by community sources, as discussed in chapter 8.

Choosing Sources of Ascertainment   Ideally, every possible source of cases should be explored (table 6.5). This is extremely expensive, and some sources provide very few cases for the effort expended. In the Maryland survey, few cases were provided by neurologists and other relevant specialists in private practice in the community. Very few practitioners returned a stamped postal card enclosed in a letter requesting cases, and the physicians were too numerous for the survey staff to do extensive follow-up telephoning. Neurologists were telephoned, but most were unable to recall the names of HD patients they had seen. The exceptions were two neurologists who lived in pockets of high prevalence and provided information about many patients. Even if they had not been directly contacted as part of the survey, these physicians would have been discovered to be important contacts, because several patients under their care were ascertained by other sources.

County health departments were the other source in the Maryland survey that proved to be less useful than expected. They kept no diagnostic files, and the clinics maintained by the health departments focused on prenatal and pediatric care.

Nursing homes and long-term psychiatric hospitals had many patients with HD and were cooperative. However, there was considerable underreporting by these sources, either because they had no systematic diagnostic records or because HD was not specifically recorded. Reporting was dependent on the memories of nurses, physicians, and medical record librarians for the recall of names of HD patients who were resident there. About one in every five HD patients known by the survey staff to be resident in these institutions was not reported to us by the institution because of either misdiagnosis or failure of staff recall. Despite underreporting, the psychiatric hospitals were an essential resource because of their medical record archives and index of patients by surname. These records provided the names of descendants of many deceased patients, documented the family history in others, and provided names of common relatives for branches of families not previously known to be related. Medical records librarians were, thus, a vital source of information.

Discharge diagnoses from the major Maryland hospitals, including the three Veterans Administration (VA) hospitals, provided the names of many patients, but approximately one-third of them did not, in fact, have HD. Nevertheless, hospitals were an important source. Patients could be screened efficiently, because all the hospitals had computerized records and recorded HD by ICD code (the International Classification of Diseases numbering system for diagnoses). Medical records could be reviewed efficiently to screen for possible cases before requesting permission from the hospital research committee to contact a family. Within Johns Hopkins Hospital, patients' names were also obtained from the Medical Genetics Clinic. This information overlapped considerably with the hospital discharge diagnoses, but added those patients who had never been hospitalized. None of the hospital-based neurology clinics provided more than the occasional case, because they did not index patients by diagnosis.

About halfway through the survey, social workers from the Department of Social Services and other agencies serving the poor began to report cases. Even though they had not been contacted formally, these agencies had heard of the services available to HD patients through the BHDP Research Clinic and referred patients for care. Many of the black patients were found in this way. Subsequently, formal approaches were made to these agencies.

The major HD voluntary health organization, the Huntington's Disease Society of America (HDSA), through its national mailing list and that of the Maryland chapter, provided the names of many persons from HD families. Many of these persons were at risk rather than affected, but some had symptoms when examined and others had affected family members.

From time to time during the survey, public service announcements were broadcast on local radio stations, and human interest articles about HD were

Table 6.5. Cases of Huntington's Disease Identified by Sources of Ascertainment

Source	Cases Identified by Source			Cases Identified Only by Source		
	Total	White	Black	Total	White	Black
General hospital discharge dx	42	31	11	6	6	0
Johns Hopkins discharge dx	35	29	6	1	0	1
Johns Hopkins Genetics Clinic[a]	36	33	3	0	0	0
Urban medical specialists	22	14	8	8	5	3
Rural physicians	13	9	4	3	2	1
National Institutes of Health	5	5	0	1	1	0
County Health Departments	6	4	2	4	3	1
Department of Social Services[b]	16	7	9	1	1	0
State psychiatric hospitals	12	8	4	1	1	0
VA hospitals	21	16	5	9	6	3
Nursing homes	17	16	1	2	1	1
Voluntary health organizations[a]	46	43	3	8	7	1
Radio and newspaper spots[a]	28	27	1	9	6	3
Genealogic investigation of reported cases[b]	98	62	36	45	28	17

[a]Lower proportion of blacks than whites ascertained by the source.
[b]Higher proportion of blacks than whites ascertained by the source.

Table 6.6. Cases Found Using Only Inexpensive and Easily Accessible Sources and Pedigree Screening

Source	Cases Found	%	Cumulative %
Johns Hopkins Genetics Clinic	90	41	41
General hospital discharges	54	25	66
HDSA Mailing List	20	9	75
VA Hospital Diagnostic Index	12	5	80
Radio and newspaper spots	12	5	85
Other	33	15	100

published in the local newspapers. This method also resulted in the ascertainment of more at-risk persons than the more medically oriented sources.

Could a subset of the sources have been used to find all the cases? To find all cases, only one source—the Johns Hopkins Medical Genetics Clinic—could have been excluded. Although it provided many cases, they all had well-documented HD and were also known to and reported by at least one other source. However, by using the genetics clinic and only four other sources that were cooperative and inexpensive to utilize (table 6.6), along with genealogic investigation of the cases reported, we would have found 85% of the cases.

Gaining Access to Sources and Patients Found through Them   Once a survey of HD has been planned, the next step is to approach the individuals and institutions where cases are registered, in such a way that cooperation is likely. It is important to learn about the administrative structure of the institutions to be approached and their process for approving research projects. A letter describing the research and a copy of the approval notification of the university's ethics committee should be sent to the appropriate person or committee, followed by a telephone call and an offer to attend any committee meetings where the research will be discussed. In this way, any services to be offered or other advantages to the patients and families can be stressed, and questions about the research can be immediately discussed, thus avoiding misunderstandings.

It is important to agree upon procedures for contacting patients and their families. Some institutions will wish to write to the families requesting permission to release the patient's name. Others will wish to send a letter composed by the investigators. If classes of individuals such as neurologists or social workers are to be contacted, access must be gained to the appropriate mailing lists. Before sending letters to them, it is useful to arrange to speak at a meeting of their professional organizations.

Once HD patients and their families are found, it is not difficult to gain their cooperation for a survey or for other research if clinical services are offered. HD families have many needs and few physicians or social agencies have either the time or experience to provide expert help. If clinical services are not provided, the population agreeing to provide information to a survey will be biased toward middle-class families and will not likely be a representative sample of HD patients.

Summary and Conclusions

The prevalence of HD is highest in populations of western European origin, consistent with the hypothesis that most HD families originated in northwest Europe, migrating from there to other parts of the world. Two surveys, in South Africa and in Maryland, found an equal prevalence of HD in whites and mixed-race blacks. HD is probably quite rare in African and Oriental populations, but is present among these groups.

Systematic surveys of a defined geographic population have been used to estimate prevalence and incidence rates. The information can be used to estimate the need for services and to evaluate the effectiveness of a planned intervention aimed at the prevention or treatment of HD. Representative HD populations ascertained through population surveys are also needed to make accurate estimates of age at onset, duration of illness, and frequency of particular symptoms.

Community surveys are also helpful in finding HD families for research and to facilitate the dissemination of information about methods available for treatment and prevention.

7

Genetics

> When either or both the parents have shown manifestations of
> the disease, and more especially when these manifestations have
> been of a serious nature, one or more of the offspring almost in-
> variably suffer from the disease, if they live to adult age. But if
> by any chance these children go through life without it, the
> thread is broken and the grandchildren and great grandchildren
> of the original shakers may rest assured that they are free from
> the diseases. . . . Unstable and whimsical as the disease may be
> in other respects, in this it is firm, it never skips a generation to
> again manifest itself in another; once having yielded its claims,
> it never regains them.
> —HUNTINGTON, 1872

Huntington's disease is inherited as an autosomal dominant trait (figure 7.1). Therefore, males and females are equally likely to be affected; on aver- age, half the offspring of an affected parent will inherit the disorder; and affected persons will be found in many generations. The gene is completely penetrant, so every individual who is heterozygous for the HD gene will even- tually develop symptoms if he or she survives through the age of risk.

Although the gene for HD is inherited in a straightforward Mendelian fash- ion, it is a gene with many unusual and unexplained features. For example, although the gene is present from conception, the onset of illness is usually delayed until adult life. Although HD is relatively common for a single-gene condition, its mutation rate is exceedingly low. And although all affected families appear to have a mutation at the same genetic locus, they vary with respect to age-of-onset distribution, neurologic manifestations, and psychiatric symptoms. Children of affected fathers are likely to have an earlier onset than children of affected mothers. Unlike many inherited diseases, persons with the HD gene have a normal or near-normal reproductive capacity in the years before the onset of symptoms. In fact, persons with the gene have more children than do their unaffected siblings (Reed et al. 1958).

While the gene that causes HD has not yet been identified, it has been localized to the tip of the short arm of chromosome 4 by genetic linkage analysis (Gusella et al. 1983; Smith et al. 1988; Hayden et al. 1988; Youngman et al.

DEMONSTRATION OF AUTOSOMAL TRANSMISSION

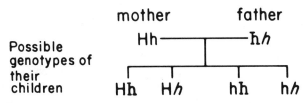

Figure 7.1. Eggs and sperm contain only one of each of the 23 pairs of chromosomes. At conception, the chromosome number is restored to 46; one chromosome of each pair is inherited from the father and one from the mother. In this example the mother has HD. Half her eggs will have the chromosome with the abnormal gene for HD (H), and the other half will have a normal gene (h). In most cases, she will marry a person without the HD gene, so all his sperm will have the normal gene (h,*h*). The parental genes at the HD locus could combine in four possible ways, as illustrated. (Note that h, ħ, and *h* are genetically identical.) Two of these combinations will result in a child with the gene for HD. Therefore, the probability of any given child's inheriting the HD gene is one-half, or 50%.

1988). Using a marker near the gene, this important discovery has made it possible to distinguish persons at risk who have a very small chance of having inherited the gene from those with a very high probability of having the HD gene. However, the marker can be used in this way only in families where several closely related members are available for study.

Finding the HD gene itself would allow the development of an accurate test (or tests, if different mutations of the gene exist) for the disease which would not depend on the availability of family members. More important, it is hoped that finding the gene responsible for HD and studying its effects will provide new ideas for rational treatment or prevention of HD.

This chapter will discuss genetic aspects of HD, including its transmission, methods used to estimate the rate of mutation of the HD gene, evidence that HD may be caused by more than one mutation, the paternal transmission effect, and genetic fitness (average number of offspring) of individuals destined to become affected by HD. A final section introduces the concept of genetic linkage analysis and its application to the search for the HD gene.

Case Example: One Man's Discovery of His Membership in a Family with Huntington's Disease

Mr. Stanley was a 33-year-old business man who had come from a poor family. His parents were divorced when he was 4 years old, and he moved to Baltimore with his mother and her second husband. He eventually obtained a college education and married a college classmate. They had two children.

Mr. Stanley had always been short tempered. As family and professional responsibilities mounted, his temper worsened and, in addition, his moods became unpredictable, so the marriage was a stormy one and eventually ended in divorce. Mrs. Stanley retained custody of the children and moved to another state.

Following the divorce, Mr. Stanley became depressed and sought help from a psychotherapist. About this time he also reestablished contact with his father, whom he found to be suffering from a neurologic condition manifested by difficulty in speaking and abnormal movements. The two did not discuss the father's symptoms, but Mr. Stanley consulted a medical textbook and concluded that his father must have Parkinson's disease. Shortly thereafter, his father died, and at the funeral Mr. Stanley met an uncle whose symptoms were similar to his father's. Although the family members at the funeral were not eager to discuss the diagnosis, an aunt eventually confided to Mr. Stanley that both his father and uncle had Huntington's disease.

Shortly afterward, Mr. Stanley made an appointment at the Johns Hopkins HD Clinic to learn more about the disease and whether he could develop it. He proved to be a member of a large well-documented kindred (figure 1.1) and could be confidently told that he was at 50% risk for HD. On examination, Mr. Stanley had no neurologic signs of HD or any other motor abnormalities. However, he gave a clear history of alternating periods of depression and hypomania, often the first manifestation of HD in his kindred.

Mr. Stanley was told that he had no motor signs of HD but that his psychiatric problems were of some concern. He contacted his former wife to inform her of the family illness. He also asked his mother whether she had known that HD was present in his father's family, but her answer was evasive.

The Mutation of the Gene for Huntington's Disease

When chromosomes are replicated in the gonads, occasional errors in copying (mutations) occur. Some mutations are harmless, but others result in an abnormal product that may be incompatible with human life or may cause an illness in the offspring who harbors it. Unless individuals with the disease are unable to reproduce, the gene is liable to be transmitted to subsequent generations.

In most genetic diseases that have been studied at the level of the deoxyribonucleic acid (DNA), there is ample evidence that the same or similar mutations have occurred repeatedly during human history. This is demonstrated when cases appear sporadically—that is, when the mutation cannot be demonstrated in anyone else in the family. New mutations causing HD, as documented by the appearance of sporadic cases, appear to be rare and are extremely difficult to prove (Shaw and Caro 1982; Quarrell et al. 1986).

Documenting a new mutation in HD requires that the following criteria be met, similar to those suggested by Stevens and Parsonage (1969).

1. The clinical manifestations must be typical for HD—that is, progressive chorea and dementia with delayed onset documented during life.
2. The patient must be demonstrated to be the offspring of his putative parents. If both parents are living, this can now be accomplished accurately by analysis of polymorphic DNA sequences of the patient and his parents.
3. The parents must be examined, be free of any symptoms of HD, and live to age 70 without symptoms.
4. The family genealogy must be extensively investigated in an attempt to discover other cases.
5. One or more of the patient's children must have inherited HD, or there must be autopsy confirmation of the diagnosis in the patient proposed as a new mutation.

These criteria are difficult to meet because symptoms are usually delayed until middle adult life, by which time the parents may be deceased. The father's identity cannot then be documented, and the parents may not have survived unaffected beyond the age of risk for HD. In the experience of the BHDP Clinic, cases reported to have a negative family history usually have a very late age at onset and affected relatives can often be found after extensive genealogic research (see figure app5.2). In the one early-onset "sporadic" patient known to the clinic whose parents were living and unaffected, the patient was demonstrated not to be the offspring of her putative father.

There are several published reports of sporadic cases of HD. Only two meet most of the criteria for establishing a new mutation in HD. The patients described by Chiu and Brackenridge (1976) and by Baraitser, Burn, and Fazzone (1983) were demonstrated to be the offspring of their parents and had typical clinical and radiologic features. The patients had not yet come to autopsy and none of their children were yet affected, but these two reports remain possible valid documentations of new mutations of the HD gene.

Several estimates of the frequency of mutations have been made from information collected in surveys (table 7.1). Two methods can be used. The *indirect*

Table 7.1. Estimates of Mutation Rate in Huntington's Disease

Study	Mutation Rate	
	Direct Method	Indirect Method
Reed and Neel 1959	5.4×10^{-6}	9.6×10^{-6}
Wendt and Drohm 1972	0	1.5×10^{-6}
Mattsson 1974	5.0×10^{-6}	0.7×10^{-6}

Note: The mutation rate is given as mutations at the HD locus per generation.

method assumes that the prevalence of HD is stable in the population. Since the results of most surveys of HD suggest that persons with the HD gene reproduce at a rate slightly below that of the general population (see below), some new mutations would be required to maintain a constant prevalence of the disease. The indirect method estimates the mutation rate required to maintain a stable prevalence, given a particular reproductive rate of HD heterozygotes relative to the general population. It should be stressed that neither of these assumptions— a stable prevalence rate of HD or a reproductive rate significantly lower than that of the population—has been unequivocally demonstrated to be correct.

The *direct method* of calculating mutation rate is based on the proportion of cases found in a representative sample who have no detectable family history of HD. The formulae for calculating the mutation rate by these two methods can be found in Mattsson (1974a). The mutation rate estimated by either of these methods is quite low, even when the above rules for documenting a new mutation are not followed.

Wendt and Drohm (1972) did follow the suggested criteria for establishing new mutations when estimating the mutation rate in cases ascertained in their survey of HD in Germany. They checked paternity in sporadic cases when parents were still living and excluded from consideration as mutations the sporadic cases where parents had died before outliving their risk for HD. After these procedures, *no* cases remained that qualified as new mutations, so the mutation rate was zero as estimated by the direct method.

Aside from the rare case reports, is there any convincing evidence for muta- tion in HD? It would be unusual, based on investigations of other genetic disorders, for a particular mutation to have occurred only once in human history. In addition to looking for sporadic cases, another approach to docu- menting new mutations is to identify HD in populations that have had no contact with western Europeans from whom they could have acquired the gene. Families with pathologically confirmed cases have been reported from Japan (Narabayashi 1973), Africa (Hayden, MacGregor, and Beighton 1980), and New Guinea (Scrimgeour 1980). While cases from these countries may well have been caused by different mutations, it has been difficult to establish that such patients have not acquired the gene from western Europeans. The Japanese have had contacts with western European traders since the fifteenth century and yet the earliest Japanese case report is from 1927, well after the time of frequent western contacts. No investigation of the Japanese HD families has explored the possibility of a western origin of the gene. Hayden (1979) believed that the African HD family found in his survey had had no contact with Europeans, but he was not able to provide documentary evidence. No blood groups were found in the New Guinea HD families that are unknown in New Guinea natives, supporting the hypothesis that the HD gene had not been introduced by Euro- peans. On the other hand, the families appear to have originated from a coastal village that was frequented by English traders in the seventeenth century.

In summary, the mutation rate in HD is low—so low, in fact, and so difficult to document that no new mutation has ever been convincingly proven. It is possible that a single mutational event may account for many apparently unrelated families with HD, at least in cases of western European extraction. Again, this would be very unusual.

When the family history is truly negative, the diagnosis of HD is likely to be wrong (e.g., Folstein et al. 1981). However, usually the family history cannot be accurately documented, so isolated cases with typical symptoms are usually attributable not to misdiagnosis or to new mutation but rather to inaccurate genealogic documentation.

Is Huntington's Disease Genetically Heterogeneous?

Genetic heterogeneity means that one genetic disorder, as defined by its clinical symptoms, can be caused by more than one mutation, although the mutation is the same in all affected members of a given family. In sickle-cell anemia, all the mutations documented in different human populations over history have occurred at exactly the same base pair in the hemoglobin gene. However, more commonly, genetic disorders are genetically heterogeneous. In *allelic heterogeneity*, a mutation at any one of several different locations within a particular gene can result in the same or very similar clinical disease. Examples include hemophilia, glucose-6–phosphate dehydrogenase deficiency, and the thalassemias (McKusick 1986; Antonarakis, Youssoufian, and Kazazian 1987). In other genetic disorders the same clinical condition may be caused in one family by a gene on one chromosome and in another family by a gene on a different chromosome. *Locus heterogeneity* is present in the lysosomal storage disorders.

Many investigators believe that HD will be shown to be like sickle-cell anemia: all cases and all families, no matter what their clinical features and regardless of their ethnic origin, will have exactly the same mutation. We now know from genetic linkage studies (see below) that all the HD families tested share the same gene locus on chromosome 4, i.e., there is no locus heterogeneity. Linkage analysis cannot detect allelic heterogeneity which is dependent upon the discovery of the gene itself. It can then be determined whether every family has a mutation at exactly the same place in the sequence of nucleotides that comprise the gene.

Many investigators have predicted there will be only one mutation for HD, because clinical symptoms are similar from one family to the next, and because all the cases could have originated from one original western European founder. However, some features differ from family to family. One possible explanation for this repeated observation is that there may be more than one abnormal allele at the HD gene locus. The most studied feature that differs significantly from family to family is the age at the onset of symptoms. Many investigators

(Wallace and Hall 1972; Went 1975, 1983; Pericak-Vance et al. 1983; Farrer and Conneally 1985; Folstein et al. 1984, 1987) have demonstrated that the age at onset of symptoms is more similar within members of a given family than it is between different families. Other studies have demonstrated that the age at onset is significantly earlier in native Africans and mixed-race blacks than it is in Caucasians (Hayden et al. 1982; Folstein et al. 1987).

Farrer and Conneally (1985) demonstrated that the age at onset of affected persons was related to the age at death of their unaffected parents and sibs, and suggested that the age at onset was influenced not by different HD alleles but by genes for aging shared by close relatives. This hypothesis implies that some aspect of an individual's genetically programed life span influences the time that HD symptoms become manifest. Persons programed for a long life would appear to have some protective factor that renders the striatal neurons more resistant to the effects of the HD gene.

The *longevity gene* hypothesis cannot explain why the age at onset should run in extended kindreds (e.g., Went et al. 1975; Faught, Falgout, and Leli 1983; Folstein et al. 1984), unless there is assortative mating for longevity (i.e., if if long-living persons preferentially marry each other) or the longevity genes were genetically linked to the HD gene. Otherwise, the familial correlation in onset should be limited to parent:sib and sib:sib similarities. In fact, careful studies by Went et al. (1983) provide convincing evidence that the age at onset and death correlations are higher within than between HD families, even when extended kindreds are considered.

The BHDP research group has demonstrated a familial aggregation of another clinical feature of HD, major affective disorder. Earlier, less systematic genealogic studies reported the same finding (Davenport and Muncey 1916; Bolt 1970). In some HD kindreds, most affected members have episodes of depression and sometimes mania. Affective disorder is not found among the unaffected relatives more often than expected from the population prevalence. In other families, major affective disorder rarely occurs in conjunction with HD (Folstein, Abbott et al. 1983, Folstein et al. 1984).

The association between affective disorder and HD is not independent of the age at onset. When HD is associated with affective disorder there is a relatively late age at onset of motor symptoms, compared with the HD population as a whole (Folstein et al. 1987). In our population of black families among whom the age at onset is early, major affective disorder (or other psychosis) is rarely seen.

The implication is that there may be two HD alleles—one associated with a relatively late onset and major affective disorder, and the other associated with an earlier age at onset and no affective disorder. This second allele would be expected to be common among blacks. An alternative possibility—more compatible with the *aging gene* hypothesis—is that when the expression of the HD gene is delayed (due to a modifying gene), different neuronal populations are vulnerable, which results in a different constellation of symptoms. A third possibility is that a given gene mutation may exert different effects in the presence of varying genetic backgrounds. Examples of this phenomenon are well known in other species but have not been systematically documented in humans.

This fascinating puzzle—whether there is more than one HD allele or not and the explanation for the variation of clinical features—will eventually be resolved by a combination of molecular genetic and neuroscientific research.

The Paternal Transmission Effect in Huntington's Disease

In addition to the family-related factor discussed above, the age at onset of HD symptoms is influenced independently by whether the HD gene is transmitted by an affected mother or an affected father. Offspring of affected fathers have an earlier onset than offspring of affected mothers (table 7.2, figure app.5.1A). Within individual affected parent-child pairs, offspring of affected mothers are likely to have an age at onset similar to that of the mother, whereas offspring of affected fathers are likely to have an age at onset earlier than the father. This observation is called the *paternal transmission effect* and was first documented by Merritt et al. (1969). Numerous investigators have confirmed the observation and excluded the possibility that it is due to ascertainment bias (Jones and Phillips 1970; Bird, Caro, and Pilling 1974; Newcombe, Walker, and Harper 1981; Myers et al. 1982; Chase et al. 1986; Folstein et al. 1987). The phenomenon is observed in all HD families, whether black or white and whether the mean age at onset within the family is early or late. The implication for genetic counseling is that the risk of developing HD decreases a little more rapidly for

Table 7.2. Relationship between Age at Onset and Sex
of the Affected Parent

| Race | N | Mean (SD) Age at Onset | | P |
		Maternal Transmission	Paternal Transmission	
White	156	45.7 (12)	38.1 (12)	.000
Black	61	40.4 (10)	32.4 (14)	.02
Total	217	44.3 (12)	36.4 (13)	.000

Source: Folstein et al. 1987
Note: When HD is inherited from the mother, age at onset of symptoms is later on average than when HD is inherited from the father. This effect of paternal transmission has been documented in numerous studies and appears to be unrelated to the average age at onset in the family or race or other clinical features.

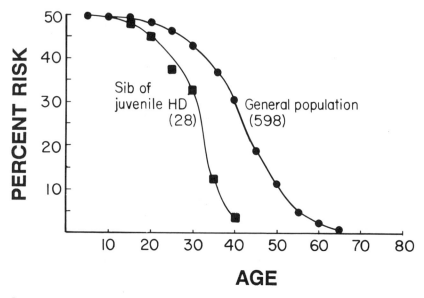

Figure 7.2. The siblings of an affected individual with juvenile-onset HD (■) are at less than 10% risk for HD by age 40, whereas the risk to sibs of adult-onset patients (●), labeled "general population," does not fall so low until age 60.

the offspring of affected fathers than for the offspring of affected mothers (figure app5.1B).

Some studies (Newcombe, Walker, and Harper 1981) suggest that juvenile cases are particularly likely after several generations of father-to-son transmission. There are some cases of child and adolescent HD inherited from the mothers, mothers who themselves had an early onset. However, as the age at onset decreases below age 20, the proportion of cases with paternal transmission increases. The phenomenon appears to be consistent for a given mating that has produced a child whose symptoms began in childhood. Their other children who become affected will have an onset of symptoms early in life (Hayden, Soles, and Ward 1985). This means that the risk is quite low that a sibling of a juvenile-onset case will develop HD after age 40 (figure 7.2).

The genetic mechanism that causes the paternal transmission effect is not understood. Clearly, it is independent of the HD gene (Farrer, Conneally, and Yu 1984; Folstein et al. 1987). Three general types of mechanisms have been proposed, but they have not been tested at the molecular level. The *mitochondrial* hypothesis has been described in chapter 5.

Another scheme was proposed by Boehnke, Conneally, and Lange (1983) in which the paternal transmission effect is accounted for by an autosomal or X-linked gene. This *modifier gene* hypothesis is somewhat less satisfying than the mitochondrial hypothesis because it requires a more complex gene effect, but the idea has not been disproven.

Gene methylation is a third possible mechanism that could account for different expressions of the same gene depending on the transmitting parent. Experiments in mice have demonstrated that some genes are more highly methylated when transmitted through a mother than when transmitted through a father (Reik et al. 1987; Sapienza et al. 1987). Methylation decreases the activity of a gene. This hypothesis implies that either the HD gene or some other gene influencing its expression is less active in individuals who have maternally transmitted HD.

In summary, the paternal transmission effect is well established in HD, but its genetic mechanism is not yet understood. Regardless of the mechanism, it is important to take the paternal transmission effect into account in genetic counseling (Hayden, Soles, and Ward 1985; Chase et al. 1986).

Genetic Fitness in Huntington's Disease

Genetic fitness in humans is usually defined as the mean family size (average number of viable offspring) of persons in some special population (e.g., HD families) compared with the mean family size of the general population of the geographic area in which the special population lives (Murphy 1978; Murphy et al. 1980).

Often the genetic fitness of persons with genetic disorders is less than that of the general population and unless new mutations of the defect occur, the frequency of the abnormal gene will gradually decrease. If the prevalence of a genetic disorder is constant in the population, any deficiencies in fitness must be equalled by new mutations. Theoretically, if the genetic fitness of persons with a particular genetic disorder were greater than that of the population, the abnormal gene would, over long periods of time, replace the normal type.

Genetic fitness of persons with the HD gene has been compared with two "normal" populations: their unaffected siblings and the general population of the geographic area from which the HD sample was drawn. Most studies have found that as a group persons with the HD gene have slightly more children than their unaffected siblings but have slightly fewer children than the general population, as shown in table 7.3.

These findings suggest that, compared with the general population, either persons with the HD gene are voluntarily limiting their family sizes to a slight extent or some aspect of their disease decreases their probability of having children. The data also suggest that the unaffected members of HD families (who do not know that they are unaffected at the time they have their families) voluntarily limit their family size to a greater extent than their siblings who are destined to have HD.

The genetic fitness of persons with genetic disease is influenced by at least

Table 7.3. Estimates of Genetic Fitness in Huntington's Disease Heterozygotes

Study	HD Patients versus Population	HD Patients versus Unaffected Sibs	HD Females versus Unaffected Female Sibs	HD Males versus Unaffected Male Sibs
Reed and Neel 1959	0.92	1.16	1.39	0.89
Wendt and Drohm 1972	—	0.96	—	—
Marx 1973	1.16	1.18	1.39	0.99
Mattsson 1974	—	0.97	1.07	0.87

Note: When correction was made for the HD heterozygotes in the sample who had not yet become symptomatic, fitness was estimated by Reed and Neel at 0.81, compared with the general population. Wendt and Drohm made a similar correction, but their fitness estimate (0.96) represents a comparison of HD heterozygotes with homozygote normal sibs. Marx and Mattsson reported results based on sibs known to be choreic at the time of the study versus all other sibs. This difference in methods probably affects estimates, with lower estimates of fitness in HD being derived when correction is made for those HD heterozygotes who are still asymptomatic at the time of study.

four factors, the first two of which are likely to operate in HD.

1. *The age at which symptoms begin.* On the average, symptoms of HD begin near the end of the reproductive years, so most persons with HD have the opportunity to complete their families before symptoms start. Once symptoms begin, they are less likely to have children (Lyon 1962). Experience suggests two reasons: first, the patient, and especially the spouse, decide to have no more children because of the burden of HD; second, there is a loss of sexual interest, first on the part of the spouse and later on the part of the patient. If symptoms begin early in the reproductive years, particularly in men, family size is curtailed. In the BHDP sample no patients whose symptoms began before puberty had children and few men whose symptoms began in their twenties had children. (The mean family size for men with onset of symptoms before age 30 was 0.5, unpublished data.)

2. *The effect of the gene on reproductive capacity.* The experience at the BHDP clinic suggests that reproductive capacity is affected in HD patients under three circumstances. First, when symptoms begin before or shortly after puberty, stature tends to be shorter than that of the unaffected sibs and puberty is delayed. Second, after a few years of illness most women experience a loss of sexual interest and men often become impotent. Third, men whose symptoms begin in their twenties have very few children. These men are often anxious and socially withdrawn during adolescence and early adult life and have had little, if any, sexual experience.

3. *Social stigma against persons with the disease.* One might expect that coming from an HD family would make it more difficult to find a marital partner who would be willing to take the risk of having to care for an ill spouse and be

willing to risk transmitting the gene to his or her children. However, some persons at risk for HD are not aware of their risk, and when they are aware they often refrain from sharing that information with their prospective spouses (e.g., Hans and Koeppen 1980). In the experience of the BHDP Clinic, even when there is full disclosure on all sides, most couples are willing to take the associated risks. In general, experience suggests that social stigma does not have much impact on reproduction in HD families.

4. *Voluntary restraint of reproduction by persons at risk.* Voluntary restraint occurs in HD families, as documented by the smaller family sizes of unaffected sibs when compared with the general population. This is less common in presymptomatic HD heterozygotes; their families tend to be somewhat larger than the families of their sibs (Shokeir 1975b). The reasons for this difference have not been studied, but clinical experience suggests that in some persons the HD gene may be manifested some years before the noticeable onset of HD, as expressed by a failure to plan, a general tendency toward disorganization, and a failure to consider the future consequences of actions.

More accurate information about the mediators of sexual behavior in HD will be needed to understand the child-bearing decisions made by persons at risk and for better approaches to genetic counseling and presymptomatic testing.

Genetic Linkage Studies in Huntington's Disease
The Definition of Genetic Linkage

Two inherited traits are said to be genetically linked when they are inherited together (rather than assorting randomly) in several members of a family. This usually occurs when the genetic loci (or sites of the genes) for the two traits lie close together on a chromosome. In medical genetics, genetic linkage is the usual method of assigning to a particular chromosome the site of a gene that causes a disease. This is accomplished by linking the disease gene to a *marker*. Many different traits can be used as markers: color vision, blood proteins, or fragments of human DNA. It is required only that the marker have a *unique locus* on a chromosome* and that the marker has more than one form, i.e., it must be *polymorphic*.

Linkage between two genetic loci is established by analyzing families in which relatives differ from each other in how they manifest the traits under study. For example, to investigate whether the gene locus for color vision (used in this case as a marker) and the gene locus for the disease glucose-6–phosphate

*It is not actually necessary to know the chromosomal locus of a marker to link it to other traits. In the past, investigators sorted traits and diseases into "linkage groups" without knowing the identity of the chromosomes on which they existed. However, at present, it is easy to establish the approximate chromosomal locus of markers and this is ordinarily known before the marker is used, or is quickly established thereafter.

dehydrogenase (G6PD) deficiency were genetically linked, it would be necessary to find a family in which some persons had normal color vision and some were colorblind *and* in which some persons in the family had normal G6PD and others had G6PD deficiency. Such a family would be polymorphic for both the disease (G6PD deficiency) and the marker (color vision).

If the two loci were genetically linked (i.e., were near each other on the same chromosome), they would be inherited together and would not assort randomly as they were transmitted through the family from one generation to the next. Figure 7.3 demonstrates a family in which a trait and a marker are genetically linked and another family in which the trait and the marker are not linked.

Linkage is ordinarily considered to be proven when the odds in favor of linkage exceed 1000 : 1. The odds are expressed as the log of the odds (LOD), so that 1000 : 1 odds is equivalent to a LOD of 3.0.

The Rationale for Genetic Linkage Studies in HD

The ultimate purpose for studying genetic diseases, such as HD, is to understand the mechanism by which the gene causes symptoms and to discover methods for prevention or treatment. One way to understand a genetic disease is to study the abnormal product made by the mutated gene. Until recently, geneticists were generally unsuccessful in finding abnormal gene products for dominantly inherited diseases such as HD. The products of dominant genes are not usually detectable because they do not circulate in the blood as do the products of recessive genes (McKusick 1986). Most dominant genes probably contain instructions for (code for) products that are built into the body's structure such as bones or membranes. Because genes for dominant disorders cannot usually be found through their products, an indirect method—genetic linkage—has been used to find the approximate location of the gene, after which attempts can be made, using the methods of molecular biology, to locate the gene precisely and synthesize its product.

Even before the gene is precisely localized, the information gained from genetic linkage analysis can sometimes be used for presymptomatic or prenatal testing for the disease. This is possible when two conditions are met: the study of many families confirms that the vast majority of families with the clinical syndrome in question show linkage to the same locus (i.e., there is no locus heterogeneity), and the marker is close to the gene so that testing is acceptably accurate.* This is the case for HD.

The usefulness of genetic linkage for finding genes for dominant disorders was limited in the past because few markers were known, and HD did not link to

---

*If the gene and marker are linked but separated by more than about one million base pairs, they will occasionally become separated at meiosis, i.e., recombine. When this happens, test results will be inaccurate. The markers currently used for presymptomatic testing are very tightly linked to the HD gene, so recombination rarely occurs.

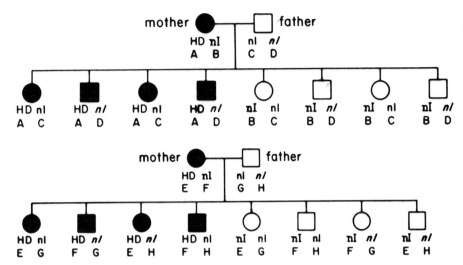

Figure 7.3. (A) The parent with HD had marker forms A and B at the marker locus being tested for linkage to HD (nl, nl and *nl* represent the normal alternative, written in different types to facilitate tracking. In all cases, the offspring who inherited HD from this parent also inherited the marker form A, and those offspring who escaped HD inherited the marker form B. Thus, the HD locus and this marker are genetically linked, i.e., exist close together on the same chromosome. (B) There is no consistency between having the HD gene and having a particular marker form from the affected parent. Some offspring affected with HD inherited marker form E and others F. Therefore, the HD locus is not linked to this marker.

any of them (Lindstrom et al. 1973; Pericak-Vance et al. 1979). It was recently discovered (Nathans and Smith 1975) that human DNA has many highly polymorphic areas which can be used as a virtually unlimited source of markers. These are neutral polymorphisms for the most part, i.e., they do not appear to cause any diseases. Many of these polymorphisms can be detected by *restriction enzymes* found in bacteria that cut (restrict) DNA at certain nucleotide sequences, often palindromes. One such nucleotide sequence is AAGCTT,* which is cut by an enzyme from the bacterium *Haemophilus influenzae*. If any one of the nucleotides in the sequence is changed, the enzyme will not cut the DNA at that point. When some individuals have a certain restriction enzyme cut site and other individuals do not, that site is said to be polymorphic in the human genome. These restriction site polymorphisms (called RFLPs, restriction fragment length polymorphisms) can be detected in the laboratory and are commonly used for genetic markers.

*DNA is made up of long strings of the deoxynucleic acids adenine, thymine, guanine, and cytosine. These are abbreviated A, T, G, and C.

The Story of the Discovery of the HD Gene Locus

One of the first dominantly inherited diseases to benefit from the discovery of the RFLP markers was HD. When HD was linked to an RFLP, only a few such probes were available and one of them was quite close to the HD locus on the tip of chromosome 4. This fortunate discovery was made by James Gusella (Gusella et al. 1983) at the Boston Huntington's Disease Center using two large HD families. One was provided by Michael Conneally at the National Huntington's Disease Roster, where the family had registered. The other was a large Venezuelan kindred around Lake Maracaibo. The origin of the family has not been precisely documented, but it is thought that the HD gene was introduced by European immigrants or sailors.

It had been one of the recommendations of the congressional commission on HD (see also chapter 1) that the Venezuelan family be documented genealogically, that its members be examined, and that blood be stored for genetic linkage study. The family was sufficiently large that if linkage were present, it alone could provide a significant LOD score to confirm linkage. Nancy Wexler undertook the administratively and politically complicated task of gaining access to the family, obtaining their cooperation, and then arranging the many trips needed to implement the field work. She was (and continues to be) assisted in the study of the Venezuelan kindred by a devoted team of clinical investigators (Young et al. 1986). The team traveled to the many small villages around Lake Maracaibo, visiting related families, examining them and collecting blood samples. The blood samples were then carried by hand to Dr. Gusella's laboratory in Boston, where the DNA was extracted and analyzed using a number of RFLP probes until linkage was detected. The results of the marker analysis were sent to Dr. Michael Conneally at the University of Indiana, who performed the formal linkage analysis and also tested for paternity. The success of such fieldwork depends on remarkable teamwork and coordination, not the least of which is transporting blood samples from the field, through U.S. Customs, and to the laboratory before the DNA deteriorates.

The time of this discovery was one of great excitement for the HD research community and the HD families. After many years of unfulfilled hopes and apparent dead ends in research a discovery now made it possible to move forward in several areas of HD research, areas that are still actively being pursued.

First, it had to be established that all HD families had a mutation at the same genetic locus. This required several years of work and the contribution of families from many clinical investigators. All the HD families tested subsequently have shown linkage to the same locus, regardless of their clinical features or ethnic origin (Folstein, Phillips et al. 1985; Bird et al. 1986; Youngman et al. 1986; Haines et al. 1986). The probe first discovered to link to HD has been localized to the distal end of the short arm of chromosome 4 (Gilliam,

Tanzi et al. 1987); more recently other probes even closer to the HD gene have been discovered (Gilliam, Bucan et al. 1987; Wasmuth et al. 1988). At this writing, at least one marker has been found that (based on limited evidence) may be within the HD gene (Hayden et al. 1988; Youngman et al. 1988; Smith et al. 1988).

The application of genetic linkage analysis to presymptomatic testing of persons at risk for HD is discussed in chapter 10.

Summary and Conclusions

Huntington's disease is inherited as an autosomal dominant trait with complete penetrance, but onset is usually delayed until adult life and the time of onset is influenced both by family membership and the sex of the transmitting parent. There is some evidence that subtle manifestations of the gene occur some years before it is possible to make a reliable clinical diagnosis. The mutation rate is low, and new mutations are difficult to document because of the late age at onset.

The genetics of Huntington's disease has fascinated clinicians and researchers for many years. On the one hand, there is a straightforward autosomal dominant pattern of inheritance and the approximate gene locus was established as soon as the necessary technology became available. However, many genetic mysteries about HD remain, including the reason for the low mutation rate, the variation of symptoms between families, the paternal transmission effect, and the delayed onset of symptoms. If these mysteries were understood for HD, they might provide clues to the mechanisms of symptom onset and pattern in other genetic disorders with similar features.

III

DIAGNOSTIC ISSUES AND PATIENT CARE

8

The Diagnosis of Huntington's Disease

> There are three marked peculiarities in this disease. 1. Its heredi-
> tary nature. 2. A tendency to insanity and suicide. 3. Its man-
> ifesting itself as a grave disease only in adult life.
> —HUNTINGTON, 1872

In principle, the diagnosis of Huntington's disease is straightforward: it is
a clinical-pathologic entity defined by involuntary movements and abnormalities of voluntary motor control which may begin at any time after infancy
but usually starts in middle adult life. Most patients also suffer from a nonaphasic dementia and emotional symptoms, particularly irritability and depression. The disease progresses gradually, with death occurring an average of 16
years after the onset. There is almost always a history of an affected parent. The
most prominent neuropathologic finding is atrophy of the head of the caudate
nucleus (Bruyn 1968).

Virtually no other condition shares this constellation of features. However,
in the Maryland survey of HD, considerable diagnostic inaccuracy was detected, as demonstrated by patients reported to the survey who did not have HD
and by the failure to report HD patients because they had been given some other
diagnosis (Folstein et al. 1986). Misdiagnosis resulted partly from physicians'
unfamiliarity with the many ways in which HD can present and partly because
of failure to take an adequate family history.

This chapter will suggest procedures by which a clinician may efficiently
acquire enough genealogic information to document the presence or absence of
HD among relatives; describe the several presentations of HD early in the
course, how its appearance changes as the illness progresses, and how the signs
and symptoms differ in black patients and in patients whose illnesses begin
either very early or very late in life; and discuss the differential diagnosis of HD
and the usefulness of laboratory tests in this regard.

Case History: The Presenting Symptoms of Early Huntington's Disease

Mr. Jones, a 28-year-old man, was referred to the BHDP Research Clinic by his
psychiatrist, who had noted that Mr. Jones had slight involuntary movements

when stressful topics were discussed. The family history of HD had recently come to light when one of Mr. Jones' siblings was diagnosed. Before this, the children had been told only that their mother died in a psychiatric hospital.

Because of his mother's illness and his father's chronic alcoholism, Mr. Jones and his three siblings were reared in a series of foster homes. During adolescence, Mr. Jones was frequently truant and was arrested twice on drug charges and possession of stolen property. He left school after the tenth grade and completed a training course in the operation of heavy equipment. He obtained steady employment, married, had two children, and gradually achieved a more stable life.

Several months before his referral to the BHDP Research Clinic, Mr. Jones' employer had referred him to a psychiatrist because of increased irritability on the job. He was also complaining of chronic back pain following an injury at work that resulted indirectly from an argument with a fellow worker. The plant physician diagnosed alcoholism because of the reports of loss of balance and irritability, although Mr. Jones denied drinking at work.

When questioned in the clinic, Mr. Jones denied any difficulties, attempting to explain away his employer's concerns. His wife, however, related that for the past year they had been having increasingly frequent arguments over minor issues and that Mr. Jones had become short tempered with the children, making unreasonable demands and taking harsh disciplinary measures. She had also noticed that he was having difficulty manipulating tools when working on his truck and that he sometimes lost his balance for no apparent reason.

On examination, Mr. Jones was a tall, well-groomed, alert man who was restless and moved about in his chair. There were frequent twitches of his face and feet. Although his answers to questions demonstrated normal comprehension and use of language and an adequate appreciation of the situation, he did not offer much spontaneous conversation and was vague about the dates and details of life events, most of which his wife supplied.

He appeared downcast and admitted to feelings of depression. On cognitive examination, he was oriented to the time and place and registered three words, but was able to recall only two of them after a distraction. He made several errors on serial sevens and could not correctly spell *world* backward.

On neurologic examination, he had mild, low-amplitude choreic movements, particularly of his face and feet but occasionally of his trunk and shoulders. These involuntary movements were more obvious when he was asked difficult questions and ceased when he was calm and relaxed. His speech was normally understandable but slightly slow and irregular in rhythm. The arrhythmia was intensified by asking him to repeat syllables quickly. There were also abnormalities of voluntary motor function. Although he was able to pursue a moving target with his eyes, he could not make saccadic eye movements quickly and he tended to move his head with his eyes. He was also unable to move his tongue rapidly from side to side, and finger-thumb tapping and rapid alternating movements were arrhythmic. His gait was normal except for difficulty maintaining his balance when walking heel-to-toe.

Given the documented family history of HD along with the patient's increasing irritability, mild clumsiness, and involuntary movements, HD was by far the most likely diagnosis. CT scan and thyroid function tests (TFTs) were carried out to rule out other possible causes for the symptoms. CT scan was read as normal and TFTs were normal. Mr. and Mrs. Jones were told that Mr. Jones suffered from Huntington's disease.

Methods of Genealogic Investigation

One neurologist with many years of experience with HD tells his students, "If you have only an hour to spend with a patient referred to rule out Huntington's disease, spend 55 minutes taking the family history and 5 minutes examining the patient" (Dr. Ira Shoulson, personal communication).

The importance of genealogic investigation in HD cannot be overemphasized. Without a definite family history the diagnosis of HD is always in doubt, and so prognosis and genetic counseling cannot be confidently provided, and the patient cannot be included in research projects. For the purpose of diagnosis, it is adequate to find one other affected relative. However, for genetic linkage and some other genetic studies and for accurate genetic counseling and presymptomatic testing, extensive genealogic documentation of many affected relatives and their ages at the onset of symptoms is needed. This section will suggest ways of collecting adequate genealogic information for these purposes.

Genealogic Notation and Taking a Family History

When taking a family history (for HD or any other medical condition), the investigator should record the information immediately, using standard pedigree notation. This notation is simple and has several advantages over recording the family history word by word. First, it is a shorthand, so the pedigree can be recorded as quickly as the informant can speak. Second, it results in accurate and unambiguous documentation. The relationships of all family members to the proband and to each other are clearly specified. Writing family histories longhand encourages a variety of inaccuracies. The notation, "Her aunt was also affected," may mean little a few hours later: whose aunt was it and on which side of the family? Use of pedigree notation also provides accurate documentation of birth dates and fewer omissions of relatives because each relative is asked about separately and according to a standard routine. Third, the use of pedigree notation facilitates patient care and genetic counseling. By asking about each family member individually, the investigator will discover other diseases that afflict the family; important family attitudes and beliefs will be revealed that will help in understanding their feelings about HD; persons who provide the family support can be recognized; and at-risk persons who may need information about HD will come to attention.

Practical Suggestions for Taking a Family Pedigree

Although it is difficult at first to arrange the pedigree on paper in an orderly way, with practice the use of standard notation to record the family history becomes routine. Books and manuals are available that explain the details of pedigree documentation (e.g., Jorgenson, Yoder, and Shapiro 1980) and its use in family studies (Krush and Evans 1984). For clinical purposes the symbols included in figure app5.2 will suffice.

Ask about each family member individually in turn, repeating the request for birth order, birth and death dates, and illnesses for each person mentioned. It has been shown empirically that the form of questioning "Did anyone have ————?" or "Did anyone have the same illness as you?" results in important omissions by the informant (Thompson et al. 1982). By asking about each person in turn, the informant's mind is focused on that person's life and more information is recalled.

It will be necessary to ask specifically about previous marriages, children born before marriage who may have been adopted away (and whose adoptive parents are almost always unaware of the child's risk for HD), and any children adopted into the family who may not be at risk. In HD families, the offspring of affected persons are often taken in by other family members at an early age and are sometimes unaware of the identity of their biological parents or their own risk for HD. Informants often omit this information unless asked specifically.

Dates of birth, age at onset of psychiatric symptoms and of motor disturbances, and age at death of closely related affected members should be recorded for use in genetic counseling. Because there is a correlation between the ages at onset within families, as described in chapter 7, this information can improve the accuracy of estimating the remaining risk of HD to family members at particular ages.

Usually, persons with HD know that someone else in the family had HD or have some information that can lead quickly to the documentation of other affected relatives. They may have been told that their father died in a psychiatric hospital or that a relative had a drunken gait or mental illness. When the patient presents with features typical of HD and available informants deny that other relatives were affected with any suspicious conditions, it is unwise to assume that their information is correct until some independent genealogic investigation has been carried out. In the rare case that a patient with typical HD presents with a convincingly negative family history, the possibility should be investigated that the patient's parents are not as reported before embarking on a medical work-up for other conditions. If paternity is documented as reported, other diagnostic possibilities should then be explored.

To explore further a family history initially reported to be negative, the investigator needs three tools: an adequate informant, a knowledge of the other disorders and symptoms for which HD may be mistaken, and access to certain medical records.

An Adequate Informant   The best informant for a family history of HD is an older unaffected family member who is in good health and who keeps in touch with the extended family. If there are no clues about which side of the family is most likely to have HD, an informant from each side will be needed. The patient and spouse can usually identify such persons. If the patient who may have HD is a young adult, a problem in family history documentation arises when one parent is well and the other died young or divorced, so contact has been lost with that side of the family. In such a situation it is useful to speak to relatives on the apparently unaffected side of the family who live in the same town as relatives on the suspected side. This strategy has frequently turned up information about affected relatives who were unknown to the patient and the unaffected parent.

The search for an adequate informant may require a series of telephone calls before a knowledgeable person is contacted. It is important to obtain permission to call each person, to protect confidentiality, and to avoid alarming the family unnecessarily. In this regard it is also useful to try to ascertain how much the person knows about HD early in the conversation to approach the subject appropriately. Finally, try to avoid discussing personal information that relatives have provided but may not wish to have shared with other family members. Informants often impulsively divulge family resentments and disagreements that are useful for the professional to know when approaching other family members but that should not be shared with them. In HD, a kindred's affected and unaffected branches may not get along; affected branches feeling angry with their bad luck and unaffected ones wishing to shun their unfortunate relatives.

The family history is often reported to be negative when a patient with clinical features of HD presents late in life, and an adequate informant may be difficult to find. The patient will likely have been diagnosed as having senile chorea, a condition presumed to be nonfamilial. However, symptoms of HD may begin after age 60 and because the age at onset tends to be similar in families, a considerable proportion of HD heterozygotes in the extended family will have died of other causes before reaching the age at which they would have developed symptoms, thus causing the family history to appear negative. Affected relatives may be found only in collateral family lines, so the investigator may need to question several informants. It is useful to begin by questioning the patient's oldest living sibling, but it may be necessary to resort to a search of medical records for relatives in prior generations. In one such family, a documented diagnosis of HD was found in the medical records of the patient's great-grandfather, who died in a psychiatric hospital (figure 8.1). In another, the

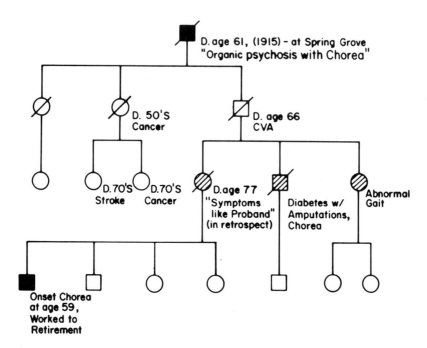

Figure 8.1. In some HD families, the onset of symptoms is ordinarily delayed until late in life. The proband in this family (designated by an arrow) knew of no other affected members. Questioning of several family members revealed other affected members, one of whom had diagnosed "organic psychosis with chorea" and had died in a psychiatric hospital.

(then mildly) affected patient returned to his hometown and questioned elderly friends of his father, who recalled that the father had had a drunken gait during his later years. In a third family, informants described elderly relatives who currently had mild involuntary movements but had not sought medical attention.

Symptoms and Diagnoses to Ask About   Once an adequate informant is found, he or she may immediately report other affected relatives. Others will know about other affected persons but be reticent about disclosing the information because of family pressures to maintain secrecy. If the immediate diagnostic dilemma and the importance of accurate diagnosis for the patient are explained, the informant will usually be willing to speak.

Other informants will never have heard the term *Huntington's disease* and it will be necessary to explain its features. Informants may recall irregular jerky movements, a drunken gait, trouble with memory, or emotional symptoms. They may be aware that a family member died in a nursing home or psychiatric hospital, retired early from work, had a drunken gait, committed suicide, had St. Vitus' dance, schizophrenia, senility, Parkinson's disease, or multiple sclerosis, all conditions for which HD is commonly mistaken (Folstein et al. 1986). Some informants will initially describe affected relatives simply as nervous.

Obtaining Medical Records   If no other affected family members are known, medical records can be requested for any relatives with histories or diagnoses that suggest HD. Such medical records frequently contain a description of the patient's clinical features that is adequate to make the diagnosis of HD even though that diagnosis was not made at the time.

Other affected family members may often be found by a systematic search of the records of the hospital in which the patient is being evaluated or in the larger general and psychiatric hospitals in the area. By supplying the names of suspect family members, preferably with birth names and dates of birth, to the medical record librarians along with signed permission to release records, any family members who had been seen in that hospital can often be found. It is wise to telephone the record librarian at the time the request for records is sent, to explain the importance of a careful search.

The construction of very large pedigrees for research purposes utilizes essentially the same process, but some additional methods are also useful. Suggestions for this type of genealogic research are contained in appendix 3.

Family History for Adopted Children   During the course of clinical and investigative work in the BHDP, several adopted children have presented with possible Huntington's disease, and numerous children at risk for HD have been reported by their families to have been adopted away. Adoption is fairly common in HD families, especially if the mother has become affected while her children are young. Adopted children pose serious diagnostic problems to physicians. The presentation of HD in children is unusual, and diagnosis may be difficult without knowledge of the family history.

Adopted children and adoptive parents have the right of access to certain information about the child's biological parents. The family should contact the adoption agency and explain the need for information about HD. The agency is required to check its own records for relevant information. If nothing is recorded, the agency is obligated to attempt to reach the biological parents or some of their relatives to investigate the possibility of HD. Obviously, the agency personnel must be provided with enough information about HD to direct their search. Sometimes children from the same HD family have been adopted by several different families, and the request for information about one affected offspring has often prompted the agency to contact other adoptive parents to inform them that their adopted child is at risk.

When the BHDP Research Clinic staff discovers at-risk children who have been adopted away, either in the context of clinical or research work, we request permission from the biological family to contact the adoption agency (see also Omenn, Hall, and Hansen 1980). The adoption agency is sent material about HD and encouraged to inform adoptive parents of their children's risk. This gives the adoptive parents the opportunity to decide on the best way of informing their children.

If the adoption was an unofficial one, the process may be more difficult, and the steps taken depend on how much the adoptive parents know about the biological parents.

The Variable Presentation of Early Huntington's Disease

Probably the most important reason for misdiagnosis of HD is that the early signs and symptoms can vary from motor restlessness to slight ticlike jerks, tremor, rigidity, irritability, depression, hallucinations, apathy, or memory loss. Up to half the patients present with only cognitive or emotional symptoms (Bickford and Ellison 1953; Brothers and Meadows 1955; Chandler, Reed, and DeJong 1960; Heathfield 1967; Bolt 1970; Mattsson 1974b). If patients presented in a characteristic and predictable way, clinicians would be prompted to ask about HD when taking the family history. It may not be possible to improve diagnosis in the community even with a specific diagnostic test, because the main problem is that HD often does not come to mind unless the patient volunteers that HD runs in the family. The presenting signs and symptoms suggest many other diagnoses that are much more common than HD, and, in the absence of a positive family history, much more likely explanations for the symptoms reported.

However, when there is a positive family history, HD is by far the most likely explanation for the symptoms listed above (discussed in chapters 2–4 and summarized in the following sections). It should be emphasized that *only one* of these signs or symptoms *or any combination of them* may be seen in patients presenting at or near the time the illness begins.

Involuntary Movements: Chorea, Motor Restlessness, Tremor, and Myoclonus

In families where the risk for HD is well known, involuntary movements are usually noted first by relatives and may lead to consultation with a physician with the foreknowledge that the patient is affected. However, in most cases, involuntary movements are not the cause for complaint and patients consult a physician because of other symptoms that have resulted in a change in the patient's ability to function at home or at work.

The most common involuntary movement seen in HD is chorea. Early in the illness it is usually confined to the distal musculature (fingers, feet, or facial muscles) and is of low amplitude. Some families say that mild twitches have been present for years before the actual onset of symptoms that interfere with functioning. These long-standing involuntary movements are usually relatively stereotyped in location and the family may interpret them as tics. Because tics are relatively frequent in the population, these stereotyped movements alone should not be used to make a diagnosis of HD.

While chorea usually begins distally, it can occur in virtually any location (face, shoulder, or abdominal muscles). Truncal chorea sometimes causes the patient to seek medical attention for backache.

In the early stages of the illness, involuntary movement may be present only when the patient is stressed, as when agitated by some mental task such as an arithmetic exercise or in the anxiety of initially greeting the physician. Patients can sometimes suppress the movements while in the physician's presence, although spouses frequently report restless movements in bed, uneven pressure on the accelerator of the car, or involuntary movement during anger or excitement.

Perhaps equally common as chorea in early HD is motor restlessness. These movements appear to be voluntary and are not particularly jerky. The patient gesticulates more than usual and appears to be uncomfortable in the chair, frequently changing positions. Persons without experience in examining HD patients may not identify these restless movements as abnormal and simply comment that the patient seemed ill at ease. While such motor activity is not in itself diagnostic of HD, other aspects of the history and formal neurologic examination may support the diagnosis.

Occasional patients have other kinds of involuntary movements, tremor and myoclonus. These are characteristic of juvenile-onset cases and are usually associated with severe bradykinesia and increased tone. However, tremor and myoclonus can be seen in adult-onset HD and in combination with normal or even decreased muscle tone. They are particularly common in black HD patients.

Abnormalities of Voluntary Movement

In early Huntington's disease, the abnormalities of voluntary movement amount to mild clumsiness, which might not cause concern unless the person knows of his risk for HD. Frequently there is difficulty with rapid, rhythmic movements. Patients are unable to move their tongues rapidly and rhythmically from side to side and they cannot tap their forefingers to their thumbs quickly and rhythmically. There are similar problems with rapid alternating movements of the hands. The gait is usually normal except when the patient tries to turn on a pivot, military fashion, or to walk heel-to-toe (tandem gait); patients maintain balance with their outstretched arms and suddenly sidestep to avoid loss of balance. As the patients are observed moving about the clinic there may be a gracelessness in their movements and, as they converse with the examiner, they may assume slightly awkward or dystonic postures.

Clumsiness may also be elicited in the history. Patients or family members may have noticed a change in handwriting; trouble using tools such as wrenches, screwdrivers, and hammers; difficulty with sewing or fine needlework; or tripping on the stairs. This sort of clumsiness is often discounted as within normal range by examiners who are unfamiliar with HD. Nonetheless, when this pattern of clumsiness is seen in someone at 50% risk for HD, for whom the findings represent a change, and in the absence of any other explanation, it is probably an early manifestation of the disease.

Certainly, a single neurologic sign cannot be used in isolation to make a diagnosis of HD, and, in the general population, orthopedic conditions, arthritis, and other peripheral and central neurologic conditions are overwhelmingly more common than HD and would be the likely explanation.

When examining a person at risk for HD, it is useful to document minor abnormalities of involuntary and voluntary movement in such a manner that they can be quantified and summed. The BHDP's quantified version of the clinical examination of the motor system (the QNE in appendix 1) can be used for this purpose. In a series of normal controls no adult scored more than four points, while HD patients had higher scores. Such a scored version of the clinical neurologic examination provides a useful way to keep track of minor motor signs, and it also allows the physician to track patients longitudinally and document any changes in performance.

Cognitive Symptoms

The degree of cognitive difficulty in early HD is highly variable. Occasional patients, especially those whose symptoms begin late in life, suffer little change in cognitive function for a number of years after onset. Usually, however, diminution of cognitive speed and efficiency and minor memory trouble are among the first signs of illness noticed by the patient, family, or employer.

The family may complain that the patient cannot give an immediate answer to a factual question, seems unable to make decisions, forgets domestic chores, plans and prepares meals poorly, and omits some elements of a sequential task. The problems with speed and efficiency are particularly evident in employed patients. They become disorganized when their workload is heavy and feel unable to set priorities. Many patients complain of being unable to recall familiar dates and the details of life events upon demand.

When the patient first presents, cognitive difficulties may be detected during history-taking. The patient may be vague about past medical illness, omitting some altogether. On examination, those patients with early HD who have cognitive decline will have prominent trouble in recalling words that they learned earlier in the examination and in doing mental arithmetic, but language comprehension and grammatical usage will be preserved.

Emotional Symptoms

Many patients with HD first consult a physician or other health care professional because of a "nervous condition." Motor and cognitive symptoms may or may not be present at this time, but when emotional symptoms are the only ones appreciated by the patient and the family doctor, a psychiatrist is usually consulted. The most common emotional symptoms early in the illness are irritability, anxiety, and depression.

Irritability is manifested in the home and at work. Patients are rarely irritable in the clinic and may deny being so. However, the spouse may divulge the patient's outbursts only when the patient is not present. Other patients are extremely anxious when they first present with HD. They appear nervous, jumpy, and wide-eyed. They have sweaty palms and are easily disconcerted by questions and tasks that they should find easy. Although HD patients have numerous reasons for anxiety, they seem particularly vulnerable to becoming anxious when under seemingly minor stress.

Depression is the other common presenting emotional disorder in HD. It may begin several years before motor signs are present and is generally episodic even if untreated. The symptoms include a dysphoric mood accompanied by sleeplessness, particularly early morning awakening; loss of appetite and sexual interest; loss of interest in activities; and difficulties in making decisions. Some patients have depressive delusions or suicidal thoughts. Manic episodes, though usually brief, can occur.

The Presentation of Juvenile Huntington's Disease

About 9% of the time (Bruyn 1968), HD becomes symptomatic before the age of 20 years. Patients whose symptoms begin before age 20 usually have an affected father, and occasionally the child's symptoms begin before the father's do (Merritt et al. 1969). The diagnosis of HD is difficult in prepubertal children because chorea is frequently absent. If the illness begins in late adolescence, the choreic form is more common.

Children presenting with HD usually have a history of satisfactory scholastic achievement followed by a gradual decline in learning and by difficulty in completing assignments (Kosky 1981). In young children a change in handwriting skills may be mentioned by the teacher. When symptoms begin during adolescence, the family may first attribute them to developmental conflicts.

School authorities may suspect drug abuse, because the patient seems slow and inattentive. Even in families where HD is known, the family may not appreciate that the child has HD because of the absence of chorea.

Eventually, bradykinesia and an awkward gait lead to referral to a neurologist. When examined, the child will be slow in all areas: motor performance, speech, and response time. Cognition, as tested by simple screening tests, is often surprisingly good, provided the patient is given plenty of time to reply. However, school performance and performance on more complex cognitive tasks are severely compromised. There may be tremor or myoclonus, but rarely chorea or motor restlessness, in children presenting before puberty. The patient sits *too* still in the chair. In contrast to the atypical and infrequent involuntary movements of juvenile HD, abnormalities of voluntary movement are typical and severe and usually quite obvious by the time the patient presents to a neurologist or other HD specialist. The ability to move the eyes voluntarily is always severely compromised; speech is slow, scant, and often low in volume. Fine motor tasks are performed very slowly, the gait is widely based and stiff-legged (often described as spastic), and patients are rarely able to tandem walk. Unlike patients with choreic HD, patients with the rigid form sometimes derive temporary benefit from L-DOPA (e.g., Jongen, Renier, and Gabreels 1980).

One juvenile-onset patient (see figure 6.1) initially presented to her pediatrician with growth failure. The standard evaluation for short stature revealed no abnormalities, but her height and weight, initially normal in early childhood, had fallen well below the third percentile by age seven. She continued to grow very slowly and at age 15 is still prepubertal. Although no other case has been so striking as this patient, most of the affected children and early adolescents examined at the BHDP Research Clinic appear to be noticeably shorter than their unaffected siblings at the same age.

Patients with juvenile onset may have epileptic seizures later in the course, particularly when the onset is before puberty (Bittenbender and Quadfasel 1962; Green, Dickenson, and Gunderman 1973; Jongen, Renier, and Gabreels 1980). Seizures have been occasionally reported in persons with young adult onset (Kereshi, Schlagenhauff, and Richardson 1980).

The Presentation of Huntington's Disease in Blacks

During the course of the Maryland HD survey, 61 black patients with HD were found (Folstein et al. 1987), and several others have since been examined at the BHDP Clinic. Examination of this unbiased survey-based sample has led us to conclude that black HD patients often present very much like individuals with juvenile onset even when their illness begins during adult life. The age-at-onset distribution for blacks is significantly younger than that of whites, and there is a greater proportion of juvenile-onset cases (table 8.1). The few patients whose symptoms have begun after age 45 have a fairly typical choreic presentation.

Table 8.1. Race-Specific Age at Onset of Motor Signs

	White	Black	Total	P
Age at onset (SD)	42 (13)	36 (13)	40 (13)	.008
Cases with onset < 20 years (%)	8 (6)	7 (11)	15 (8)	.09
	(N = 156)	(N = 61)	(N = 217)	

Source: Folstein et al. 1987.

Most blacks present with complaints about their gait and when examined have hyperreflexia with increased tone, sometimes with cogwheeling, but usually they have "lead-pipe" hypertonia with increased tone throughout the range of joint motion. Most blacks also have severely impaired saccadic eye movements. They seldom suffer from major depression or other psychotic features, but their cognitive impairment is not obviously different from whites. Some patients have mild chorea, but akinesia is more common, with or without tremor or myoclonus. The course of illness is not different from that of Caucasian patients, although neuropathology can sometimes be unusual (Zweig et al. in press). As described in chapter 6, there is considerable genetic and neuropathologic evidence that these patients do have HD.

The Presentation of Huntington's Disease with Onset in Old Age

Symptoms begin after age 55 in about 10% of patients. Late-onset patients usually have prominent chorea and, initially, have relatively less difficulty with fine motor control. They are less likely to be irritable and aggressive but are more often depressed. Their cognition is usually well preserved and many can continue to work, even in professional employment if the tasks are familiar, for several years after the onset of obvious chorea. Limited evidence suggests that symptoms progress more slowly when the onset is late (Myers et al. 1985).

Diagnosis can be difficult here as well, even though their presentation is much more typical of HD. First, some physicians believe that HD cannot begin at age 60 or 70 and do not consider the possibility. Second, there can be coexisting vascular disease that may provide another explanation for the symptoms. Third, most patients are well preserved cognitively and are unlikely to exhibit personality change. Fourth, the family history is often reported to be negative. The combination of very late-onset chorea with a negative family history and preserved cognition and personality are the diagnostic criteria for "senile chorea." Involuntary movements in old age have numerous causes, but for half the elderly choreic patients detected in the Maryland HD survey whose symptoms began at age 60 or later, other affected family members were documented by an extensive exploration of the family. Some examples were described earlier in this chapter and in chapter 6.

The Natural History of Huntington's Disease

The Progression of Symptoms

The full HD syndrome is usually well developed within three or four years of the onset regardless of whether the patient initially presented with motor, cognitive, or emotional symptoms. Although there are exceptions to the general pattern, the typical patient will sometime during the first third of the 15- to 19-year course have a functionally disabling cognitive decline, have chorea that is easily observable but not functionally incapacitating, and exhibit mild motor incoordination, tripping, and falls, but remain capable of complete self-care. Nearly all patients at this stage of the illness are able to care for themselves with limitations mainly attributable to a lack of initiative rather than incapacity. About 30–40% of patients by this stage will have had one or more periods of depression, either before or after the onset of other symptoms (see table 4.2).

Signs and symptoms that are characteristic of the middle stage of HD usually begin five years or more after the initial onset. The symptoms are similar in kind to those of the first few years but are more severe and begin to interfere with function. Irritability and apathy can appear or become worse if already present; cognition becomes more globally impaired; chorea is of higher amplitude and more constant; and motor incoordination begins to interfere with clarity of speech, self-care, cooking, housekeeping, and making home repairs. Patients become more set in their routines and are increasingly self-centered. They are readily frustrated by their increasing failures to perform and by their increasing inability to communicate effectively because of dysarthria and an inability to speak fluently. Most patients can still be left unattended during the day during this middle period, but two new symptoms appear that makes this risky— difficulty with swallowing and increasingly frequent falls.

Some patients change very little during this middle period and appear to reach a plateau. Decline is still occurring, but changes in function are so gradual that families and caregivers perceive little change over the short term.

The late stage of HD often seems to begin suddenly even though serial measures of neurologic state and activities of daily living have demonstrated a gradual decline. It seems sudden because the family and other caregivers are frightened by a life-threatening choking spell or serious fall and suddenly realize that the patient now needs constant supervision and help with eating and walking. Gradually, the patient spends more and more time in bed, finding it too tiring to maintain an upright posture. It is during this period, after 10 or more years of illness, that the death rate rises, usually from suffocation or pneumonia resulting from aspirated food.

In this late stage of HD, physical incapacity overtakes and replaces emotional symptoms as the most serious problem for caregivers. Although involuntary movements may gradually subside during these years, the voluntary motor impairment worsens. Advanced patients often have increased tone and contractures, and they eventually become virtually immobile and mute except when they are greatly excited. One family member described her mother as being locked inside her body. Despite the extreme limitations in the capacity to respond, many advanced HD patients give evidence of continued ability to comprehend their surroundings. When highly excited (by seeing a new family car or a new grandchild, for example), patients may suddenly blurt out an appropriate verbal response or try to take some socially appropriate action. This is very different from patients with Alzheimer's disease, who neither recognize nor respond to family members. Toward the end of life, HD patients may cease to recognize their family. This often occurs after repeated bouts with pneumonia or hypoxia. If patients survive to this stage, the cause of death is usually intractable pulmonary infection.

The Diagnosis of a Case That First Comes to Attention Late in the Disease

Consultants are occasionally asked to see an undiagnosed patient in a long-term care hospital who is rigid, immobile, mute, and generally unresponsive. The differential diagnosis is fairly extensive but in one case series of such hospitalized patients who were selected for being in a persistent vegetative state, Huntington's disease accounted for 13.5% of the sample. Alzheimer's disease was the most common diagnosis (Walshe and Leonard 1985). Autopsy is probably the only way to reach a diagnosis for such a patient if no family information is available, although CT scan can be helpful if the patient can cooperate.

During the Maryland HD survey, several such undiagnosed patients with advanced HD were ascertained in the process of screening families of known cases. Previous consulting neurologists, some of whom had been told of the family history of HD, had been unwilling to entertain that diagnosis because the patients had no chorea and because they had long tract signs, that is, hyper-reflexia with clonus and extensor plantar responses. Most consultants see HD patients in clinic settings when their signs and symptoms are more typical, but rarely have the opportunity to observe their deterioration to the rigid, achoreic state.

The Duration of the Illness and Causes of Death

The duration of the illness, from the first detectable motor symptoms to death, ranged from 1 to 40 years in the patients from the Maryland survey who have died (see figure 1.3). The mean duration of illness was 15.9 years. These estimates are subject to the limitations that derive from the difficulty in dating the age at onset. First, the onset is insidious and the early signs are often not attributed to illness, so it is difficult for family members to recall exactly when the illness began. Second, age-at-onset distributions are often derived from cross-sectional survey data, and patients who have died after only a few years of illness will be underrepresented in such samples (Chase et al. 1986). Based on estimates derived from cross-sectional samples, 15 years is the most frequently published figure for the mean duration of illness (Reed et al. 1958; Bruyn 1968). However, data from the National HD Roster, which is not based on a cross-sectional sample, gave an estimated mean duration of illness of 19 years (Conneally 1984) and may be a more accurate estimate.

Causes for the variability in the duration of illness in HD are easier to understand than those for the variability in the age at onset. There are risks for death at all stages of the illness. Early in the illness, some proportion of patients commit suicide. This occurs most often during an episode of untreated depression, but an occasional patient decides, based on observation of affected relatives, that he does not want to live out the course. So-called passive suicides, falls from high places and automobile accidents, also contribute to early deaths of some patients.

After the first 8 to 10 years of illness, depending on how fast the illness progresses, patients are at risk for death from truly accidental falls that result in subdural hematomas, and from choking on food. Whether these events occur depends on how much independence the patient insists upon and whether the patient is closely supervised. Because of financial considerations, many patients are left alone for substantial portions of the day. If falls and choking are avoided and if family members choose to have a feeding gastrostomy inserted when dysphagia becomes severe, patients can survive for many years. Some patients with gastrostomies live for several years after they can no longer perform any voluntary movements and are completely mute and unresponsive.

One other reason for survival beyond 20 years is an unusually slow progression of illness. In the Maryland survey those patients who had survived for more than 20 years after onset were in some ways better preserved than other patients with shorter durations. As compared to the rigid, mute state of most very advanced patients, they could all speak, most could walk, and chorea still predominated (Folstein et al. 1986).

The Differential Diagnosis of Huntington's Disease

The differential diagnosis of HD theoretically includes all conditions that have abnormal involuntary movement (chorea, athetosis, dystonia, tremor, tics, or myoclonus); abnormalities of voluntary movement (incoordination, bradykinesia, ataxia, or apraxia); or abnormal mental states (dementia, depression, mania, hallucinations, anxiety, or irritability). Rarely, injury to peripheral nerves is reported to cause involuntary movements (Schott 1986).

The various disorders that are usually included in the differential diagnosis of HD are listed in table 8.2. They are described in standard neurology texts (e.g., Adams and Victor 1985; Rosenberg 1980; see Bruyn 1986 for a description of chorea acanthocytosis). Most of these conditions are seldom confused with HD, even though they share one or more symptoms, because they are even rarer

Table 8.2. Differential Diagnosis

Movement disorders	Dementias
Parkinson's disease	Alzheimer's disease
Wilson's disease	Creutzfeldt-Jacob disease
Dystonia musculorum deformans	Pick's disease
Sydenham's chorea	Emotional and perceptual disorders
Chorea of pregnancy (or birth control pills)	Manic-depressive illness
	Schizophrenia
Hyperthyroid chorea and tremor	Abnormal behaviors
Benign familial chorea	Alcoholism
Friedreich's ataxia and other olivo pontocerebellar ataxias	Antisocial personality disorder
Strokes of the basal ganglia	
Hallervorden-Spatz disease	
Adult-onset lipid storage diseases (e.g., Kufs' disease)	
Systemic lupus erythematosus	
Tertiary syphilis	
Chorea with acanthocytosis	
Fahr's disease (familial idiopathic calcification of the basal ganglia)	
Multiple sclerosis	

than HD (for example, only twelve families with benign familial chorea have been reported; Pincus and Chutorian 1967; Suchowersky et al. 1984) or have obvious differentiating features.

The probability of a general practitioner's needing to make the diagnosis of HD is small, so it is not often included in his differential diagnosis of the usual presenting complaints of HD unless the patient or family volunteers that HD runs in the family. He will likely refer patients with such complaints to a specialist based on the predominant symptom or sign. The differential diagnoses considered by the consultant specialist depend on whether he ordinarily sees patients with movement disorders, dementia, or emotional disorders.

When cases of HD were requested from both general practitioners and specialists during the Maryland survey, each patient referred was examined by a team of specialists including neurologists and psychiatrists. The disorders that were mistakenly called HD included only the more common conditions (table 8.3) from the comprehensive list of possible causes of chorea, dementia, and emotional disorder.

Genealogic investigation of families ascertained through a correctly diagnosed relative made it also possible to detect some patients with HD who had been given other diagnoses. Again, their diagnoses reflected their predominant presenting complaints and tended to be conditions that are more prevalent than

Table 8.3. Other Diagnoses Given by the Maryland Survey to Patients Reported
as Huntington's Disease

Diagnosis	N	Diagnosis	N
Tardive dyskinesia	8	Familial dystonia	1
Alzheimer's disease	4	Syphilis	1
Psychosomatic disorders	3	Progressive supranuclear palsy	1
Stroke	3	Multiple sclerosis[a]	1
Other dementias	2	Benign familial chorea	1
Mental retardation with chorea	2	Friedreich's ataxia	1
Parkinson's disease	1	Postencephalitic parkinsonism	1
Occult hydrocephalus	1		

Note: N = 31, or 15% of the 212 cases reported.
[a]This patient's grandparent had HD.

Table 8.4. Other Diagnoses Given in the Community to Patients Meeting the Maryland Survey Criteria
for Huntington's Disease

Diagnosis	N	Diagnosis	N
Alcoholism	7	Other psychiatric diagnosis	3
Mental retardation	4	Senile chorea	2
Movement due to trauma	3	Parkinsonism	1
Schizophrenia	2	Growth failure	1
Affective disorder	1		

Note: N = 24, or 11% of the 217 patients meeting the criteria.

HD (table 8.4). Mattsson (1974b) investigated whether the type of specialist first consulted affected the misdiagnosis rate and found that it did not. Psychiatrists and neurologists were equally likely to miss the diagnosis.

A discussion of the extensive differential diagnosis of HD is beyond the scope of this book and can be found in standard texts of neurology and psychiatry. However, it may be useful to mention two conditions that have provided particularly difficult diagnostic problems, because they are relatively frequent and have clinical features that overlap substantially with those of HD: subcortical stroke and tardive dyskinesia.

Stroke

Patients with subcortical strokes can present with symptoms almost indistinguishable from those of HD and may even follow a course of illness typical for HD (Folstein et al. 1981; Richfield, Twyman, and Berent 1987). Their symptoms can include chorea, dementia, and affective disorder. The family history will be negative for HD, although it may be positive for vascular disease. The diagnosis can usually be made by computed tomography (CT) or magnetic resonance imaging (MRI) scan, which usually reveals a subcortical stroke or multiple lacunar infarcts.

Tardive Dyskinesia

The diagnosis of HD is frequently entertained for patients with tardive dyskinesia (TD), and some HD patients are misdiagnosed as having TD, although this was not observed in the Maryland survey cases. Patients with TD often have a family history of psychiatric disorder, which is also commonly reported by family members of HD patients. Sometimes HD families know only that a parent died in a psychiatric hospital or committed suicide. TD patients may have psychiatric features virtually identical to those seen in HD, and patients with both disorders frequently have a history of phenothiazine use. Finally, the involuntary movements seen in TD can be identical to those seen in HD patients. Although the involuntary movements of TD are usually limited to the mouth and face, they can involve the limbs.

However, while TD patients can sometimes have quite severe involuntary movements, they seldom have abnormalities of voluntary movement such as clumsiness, gait disturbance, and dysarthria. When they do have voluntary motor impairment, it is quite mild relative to that seen in HD patients (David et al. 1987).

The Diagnostic Evaluation for Huntington's Disease

In most cases when the presentation is typical and the family history is clear, the diagnostic evaluation need only include a careful family history, documentation of insidious onset and a gradual worsening of symptoms, and a neurologic examination. Persons at risk for HD can, of course, have other conditions, but for the overwhelming majority of persons with a positive family history and typical symptoms no other cause for the symptoms will be found.

Laboratory tests should be carried out to eliminate other more common conditions such as stroke or hyperthyroidism, but the results of such tests can be misleading. Occasionally, hyperthyroidism can cause chorea, but patients with HD also have abnormalities on tests of thyroid function more often than expected (Murthy, Rosen, and Babu 1977). CT scans are commonly read as normal early in the disease, and a normal scan may lead an inexperienced clinician falsely to exclude the possibility of HD. Later in the illness, CT scans are usually abnormal, but the cortical atrophy and enlarged ventricles may not suggest a specific diagnosis and may be read by the neuroradiologist as generalized atrophy with ventricular enlargement.

Only about 5% of the cases in the Maryland survey sample had typical symptoms along with a family history that was either negative or could not be obtained because of unknown paternity or adoption. This situation is likely to occur much more frequently in clinical practice, because the range of cases seen is wider and detailed genealogic documentation may not be practical. When the report of a negative family history is verified by extensive investigation, when adoption records cannot be obtained, or when the family history is complicated by unknown paternity, a thorough diagnostic evaluation for other causes of the symptoms is indicated.

Probably the most important first step in the evaluation of a case with a negative family history where both parents are living is to investigate the possibility that the father's identity is not being correctly reported. If paternity is validated or cannot be tested, a medical evaluation for other neurodegenerative disorders is in order. EEG (to check for the slowing typical of Alzheimer's disease), CT scanning (to investigate strokes or calcification of the basal ganglia), lumbar puncture (including tests for syphilis and multiple sclerosis), screening for thyroid and other autoimmune disorders and for adult-onset lipid storage diseases (Kufs' disease), and a careful cognitive examination to screen for aphasia and other signs of cortical dementia will usually clarify the diagnosis. Although the disorder is exceedingly rare, most clinicians will test ceruloplasmin and examine the eyes for the Kayser-Fleischer rings of Wilson's disease, because it is a treatable disorder. Occasionally, it is necessary to wait for autopsy to confirm the diagnosis of HD.

The Use of Various Brain-Scanning Techniques for Diagnosing Huntington's Disease

Because the diagnosis of HD can be so difficult to make when symptoms are just beginning, a number of methods have been explored in the hope of finding a biological test that is reliably and validly abnormal early in the illness. The genetic linkage test (to be described in chapter 10) is the most accurate way to accomplish this, but its use and applicability are currently limited. Quantitative analysis of CT scans and, more recently, PET scans has been explored to assess their usefulness in diagnosing patients who either are asymptomatic or have minimal symptoms.

CT scans are usually read as normal in the early years of illness, when the diagnosis could be in question. However, more quantitative methods have demonstrated that many mildly affected patients have measurements of caudate size significantly below those for age-matched controls. The ten patients selected by Hayden et al. (1986) for having normal CT scans all had values below the mean for the age-matched controls. Based on their scores on the Mini-Mental State Examination (MMSE), which ranged from 30 to 17 with a mean of 22.6, not all those patients could be said to be minimally affected.

Starkstein et al. (in press) compared age-matched controls with 13 HD patients whose durations of motor impairment was less than three years. These patients had MMSE scores ranging from 19 to 30 with a mean of 24.2, so, again, not all were minimally affected from the cognitive perspective. Bicaudate ratios for patients and controls (see figure 8.2 for definition) were significantly different at the .01 level, but there was some overlap between patients and controls. The sensitivity (the proportion of HD patients found to be abnormal on the scan) was 77% and the specificity (the proportion of controls scoring normally on the scan) was 92%. These findings suggest that CT could probably be used in restricted circumstances (as when the person being tested is known to be at 50% risk for HD) as a confirmatory test earlier in the disease than is currently the practice if age-specific norms for caudate measures were available for comparison with patients' scans.

At this writing, little information is available in the literature about the use of magnetic resonance image (MRI) scanning to diagnose HD. It clearly detects caudate atrophy in identified patients (Kozachuk et al. 1986; Simmons et al. 1986; see figure 5.6), but its use in minimally symptomatic cases has not yet been reported.

There has been considerable interest in using positron emission tomography (PET) with radiolabeled 2-deoxyglucose as a confirmatory diagnostic test for patients with mild symptoms and even for presymptomatic diagnosis. Markedly decreased striatal glucose utilization was first reported in HD patients by Kuhl et al. (1982; 1985). They reported profound hypometabolism in the caudate but not in cortex or thalamus. They further reported that the degree of caudate hypometabolism was unrelated to the severity of chorea and dementia, but they did not report how these clinical features were measured, and they clearly did not use standard tests and examinations. Young et al. (1987) examined diagnosable HD patients with slight or mild abnormalities in social function (stages I and II on the Functional Capacity Scale of Shoulson and Fahn 1979). All the patients had at least mild neurologic signs when examined according to a standard protocol, similar to the one included in appendix 1. The rate of glucose metabolism in the caudate was lower for stage II than stage I patients. Although glucose metabolic rates in the age-matched controls were significantly higher than in either stage I or II HD patients, the 99% confidence intervals overlapped substantially between controls and stage I patients. On the other hand, Hayden et al. (1986) reported on ten mildly affected patients who had had symptoms for less than five years and found no overlap in measures of caudate glucose metabolism between patients and age-matched controls. The most likely interpretation of the conflicting results among these three research groups is that they have different thresholds for diagnosis. Young and Penny have extensive experience in using a standardized protocol for examining and recording the neurologic examination of persons with and at risk for HD (Young et al. 1986), a procedure that in my experience gradually leads one to have a low threshold for the detection of neurologic abnormalities in persons known to be at risk for HD.

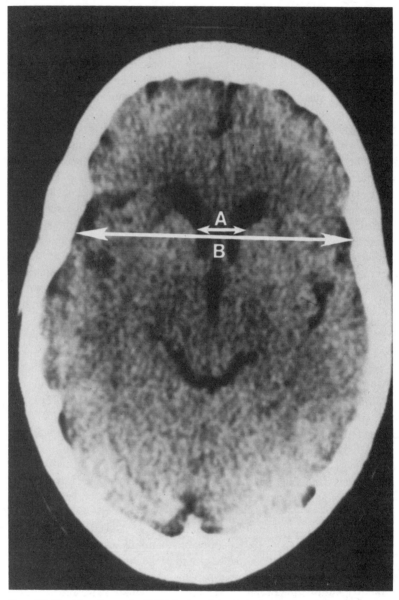

Figure 8.2. The bicaudate ratio (*BCR*) is the minimal distance between the caudate indentations (*A*) divided by the distance between the inner tables of the skull along the same line (*B*), and multiplied by 100.

The PET studies of at-risk persons claimed to be symptom free are similarly conflicting. Kuhl's group (Mazziotta et al. 1987), now using more standard methods of clinical documentation, continue to report decreased glucose metabolism rates in asymptomatic persons. Young and Penny selected their at-risk sample for having either no scoreable points on their standard neurologic examination or extremely minor signs, such as slow or dysrhythmic rapid alternating movements or slow saccades or occasional twitches that could not confidently be called choreic. All these persons had caudate glucose metabolism rates well within the normal range (Young et al. 1987).

Confirmation of the Diagnosis by Neuropathology

The diagnosis of HD is essentially based only on the observation of the characteristic clinical features in the patient and at least one other family member. Because the diagnosis implies such a grim prognosis for both patient and family, it is reassuring for the physician to have autopsy confirmation in at least one family member as evidence for a positive family history.

The characteristic neuropathologic features of advanced HD—atrophy and the depletion of neurons in the caudate nucleus and putamen—are rarely seen in other conditions and, in combination with a typical clinical course, can be confidently used to confirm the diagnosis. However, even the autopsy can cause uncertainty. The brains of patients who die within a few years of the onset will not reveal any obvious striatal pathology on routine neuropathologic examination, even though obvious clinical manifestations were observed during life. When this occurs, the clinician must weigh the evidence and occasionally should make the diagnosis even without neuropathologic confirmation. The brains of HD patients who had died early in the course of illness, which appear normal neuropathologically, reveal clear neurochemical abnormalities of the type expected (Walker et al. 1984). However, this type of examination is not ordinarily available in clinical practice.

Summary and Conclusions

The diagnosis of HD is currently based on the presence of a positive family history, plus an insidious, progressive disorder of involuntary and voluntary movement, cognition, and often psychiatric disturbance. Once the gene for HD is found, and the mutation or mutations leading to HD are established, an accurate biological test can be devised. Because HD is uncommon and because its presentation is so variable, the diagnosis is often overlooked for some years after the onset and sometimes throughout life. Diagnosis is easier if the family history is known. The differential diagnosis of HD is extensive, but the most common diagnostic errors involve conditions that are more prevalent than HD with clinical features that overlap those of HD. These conditions include subcortical stroke, tardive dyskinesia, schizophrenia, and the cortical dementias such as Alzheimer's disease. Diagnosis can be rendered with more confidence when the diagnosis in at least one family member has been confirmed neuropathologically.

9

Treatment

I have never known a recovery or even an amelioration of symptoms in the form of chorea; when once it begins it clings to the
bitter end. No treatment seems to be of any avail, and indeed
nowadays its end is so well-known to the sufferer and his
friends, that medical advice is seldom sought. It seems at least to
be one of the incurables.
—HUNTINGTON, 1872

Today there is still no treatment that can cure Huntington's disease, delay
its onset, or slow its course. Numerous experimental drug trials have been
carried out based on at least three different paradigms that reflect changing
conceptions of the pathophysiology of HD. Unfortunately, none has been
successful to date, but our ability to investigate the nervous system is improving
rapidly and there is real hope that an effective treatment will be found.

Currently, social supports and nursing interventions can improve the quality
of life for patients and their families; and medications, if carefully titrated,
monitored, and modified from time to time, can alleviate certain manifestations
of HD, particularly involuntary movements, depression, and irritability. The
medical and social resources needed to support and treat HD patients adequately are considerable and not readily available to most families. These
services are limited partly because of financial constraints but also because
physicians and other health care professionals rarely have the opportunity to see
enough HD patients and families to acquire the experience needed to develop
confident treatment plans.

One purpose of this chapter, then, is to outline recommendations for social
and pharmacologic interventions that have been helpful to HD patients and
families. These are based on experience at the Johns Hopkins BHDP Research
Clinic and on discussions with other clinicians experienced in the care of HD
patients. The chapter also reviews the rationale and outcome of some of the
experimental therapeutic trials.

Case Example: A Treatment Plan for One Patient with Huntington's Disease

Mrs. Greene was referred to the Johns Hopkins BHDP Research Clinic by her general practitioner, who had diagnosed HD based on his observation of a similar illness in her father. Her father was an immigrant whose family history could not be checked, so his diagnosis had been uncertain. Mrs. Greene was accompanied by her husband, who was distressed at the recent changes in his wife's behavior. Because Mrs. Greene's father, now deceased, was the only affected person known to the family and because his diagnosis had been in doubt, the family had never sought information about the clinical features, prognosis, or pattern of inheritance of HD.

Mrs. Greene's diagnosis of HD was confirmed based upon an examination, a review of her prior evaluations, and her father's medical records. The couple, especially Mr. Greene, had many questions about HD, which he asked in a disorganized, random way reflecting his distress. At this first visit, some information was provided to the couple about the nature of HD and its inheritance, and they were given some literature designed for patients and families. The social worker tried to focus Mr. Greene's attention on working out solutions to current problems. The most pressing problem was the effect of Mrs. Greene's symptoms on the family's domestic life. In a private discussion, Mr. Greene and the clinic social worker outlined possible arrangements for child care and housekeeping and considered strategies for presenting these arrangements to Mrs. Greene gradually, to try to gain her acceptance. One of these issues was then discussed with Mrs. Greene, who, after initially denying any need for help, agreed to a part-time housekeeper.

Two weeks later a second visit was arranged to assess Mrs. Greene's response to her diagnosis and the planned household changes and to provide any necessary support or medication. The social worker repeated some information that the couple did not recall from the first visit and raised with the couple the risk of HD to Mrs. Greene's siblings and children. They discussed how best to inform them about HD. The household was still in some chaos, so domestic issues were again discussed. Mr. Greene was put in touch with the husband of a patient whose social and domestic situation was similar. He was also referred to the local chapter of the Huntington's Disease Society of America and to a professional financial planner.

After about three months' time, two more visits, and several telephone calls, the Greene family began to accept the reality that Mrs. Greene had a chronic illness and was learning to cope with its effects.

Once the issues surrounding diagnosis were dealt with, visits to the clinic were decreased to every six months to monitor Mrs. Greene's mood and motor problems and to continue to assess the need for interventions in the household. As the years passed, many issues were raised and dealt with. These included concerns about Mrs. Greene's irritability; her initial refusal at each stage of the illness to accept needed assistance; Mr. Greene's intermittent loss of patience with his wife's demands and limitations; the impact of the illness on the children's marital decisions; the need for mechanical aids for feeding, walking, and bathing; and intermittent concerns about "what will happen next" and the feasibility of continued home care.

Gradually, Mrs. Greene's siblings and children presented to the clinic for genetic counseling and concern about symptoms. Those who escaped HD were able to provide support for those who did not.

Supporting Patients and Families through the Process of Diagnosis

When a person who knows of his risk for HD begins to experience the early symptoms, his first response is often to deny them by seeking alternative explanations: "Everyone gets depressed once in a while"; "I've always had a short fuse"; "Anyone would have fallen in that situation." When family members suggest seeing a physician, patients may refuse or procrastinate. To face a diagnosis of HD requires courage and entails the loss of hope associated with the 50–50 possibility that one may yet escape HD. Spouses occasionally call for advice about how to convince the patient to accept a clinic appointment. If diplomacy and a supportive approach fail, the spouse may need to threaten the patient with loss of support to ensure a clinic visit. While such tactics are to be avoided when possible, having a diagnosis can be essential to the well-being of the patient and the family.

Once undiagnosed patients have agreed to attend clinic, they usually come without further argument and are prepared for the outcome. Some will inform the physician that they know they are affected with HD. Once the diagnostic process is started, a clear answer should be provided to someone in the family as soon as the physician is confident that the illness is present. Some physicians, to delay giving such sad news, schedule psychological testing and scans and return visits months later. This delay increases the anxiety of the patient and the family as they await the inevitable. The decision about when to tell the patient (as opposed to the family) is more problematic. We often delay diagnosis when patients present in the midst of a depression until the depression has been treated. We also try to avoid giving a diagnosis to someone who is unaccompanied by a family member or close friend. Most patients experience a peculiar sense of relief at the diagnosis: it signals an end to uncertainty and to the increasingly difficult task of explaining away symptoms. Further, a diagnosis allows patients to become patients and accept care and support from their families and from health care professionals. And finally, an official diagnosis provides many patients with an opportunity to retire on disability pay from employment that has become too difficult and from which they may have been threatened with dismissal.

A minority of patients continue to deny the diagnosis after being informed of it, arguing with the physician about the interpretation of clinical findings and refusing to accept treatment or to discuss the issues surrounding diagnosis. Such patients demand proof such as a CT scan (which is unhelpful in confirming the diagnosis early in the course) or "the test" (the presymptomatic test, which is not usually appropriate for confirming a clinical diagnosis, as discussed in chapter 10). Such patients are frequently unwilling to accept treatment for symptoms that may be present.

Occasionally, families request that a patient not be told of the diagnosis or the patient, while willing to accept treatment for "nerves," fends off all opportunities to discuss the diagnosis. This is probably acceptable if no important life decisions (such as childbearing plans) hinge on the patient's knowledge and if the spouse is informed and can provide information to children and other relatives who need information about their risk for HD. Patients who refuse to discuss the diagnosis are almost surely aware that they are affected. Family members sometimes report overhearing such a patient discussing his illness with another affected sibling at a family gathering.

Patients should be encouraged to discuss their feelings and fears about the diagnosis. Some are concerned that their families will abandon them; others are concerned about losing their jobs; many are angry and frustrated by the loss of their future. Patients often grieve not only for themselves but also for their children, whose risks jump from 25% to 50% with the onset of the parent's symptoms.

Significant family dissension may have arisen during the time between the onset of symptoms and the diagnosis. Explaining to the patient and spouse that depression and irritability are symptoms of illness rather than reflecting a lack of feeling for the family, can help to restore trust and allow mutual support.

It is important to support the spouse during the time of the diagnosis. The spouse's reaction will depend partly on previous knowledge. Some are only too well aware of the implications of the diagnosis, having experienced the illness of other family members. Others have not even been aware of the patient's risk for HD and are completely ignorant of the clinical features of illness (Hans and Koeppen 1980). Information about the course of the illness and eventual prognosis and suggestions for restructuring finances and family life should be given gradually over several return visits as appropriate to the family's needs at the time and based on a judgment about what information they are prepared to hear. The anxiety level of both the patient and the spouse is often so high at first that they will not be able to assimilate much information, and some information may have to be repeated on several occasions. Appropriate written material, such as brochures and articles about HD, should be provided so that the family can read the information at home. Families may also request written information to send to relatives. This can be obtained from the local or national HD voluntary organization (see appendix 4 for names and addresses of national organizations; Miller 1976). It can also be helpful to put the family in touch with another family who is coping well and is willing to offer support. Such arrangements may be made by the local HD voluntary organization.

Obtaining Supports

If the family income is adequate to meet the needs of the patient and family during the prolonged course of HD, other problems and issues are usually perceived as tragic but manageable. Unfortunately, many patients become affected with HD before they have gained seniority in their jobs or accumulated much in the way of savings. Most are working families whose financial reserves in any case are modest (Tyler et al. 1982, 1983). Some supports are available.

Disability Benefits

If the patient has worked and contributed to Social Security, he will be eligible for Social Security Disability Insurance (SSDI) and any private disability insurance that may be available through the employer. Two steps must be taken to assure that the patient qualifies for disability payments when he is no longer able to work. First, the physician should try to ascertain whether job performance has deteriorated by the time of the first visit. The patient may deny job difficulty if questioned generally but admit to having been passed over for promotion, denied an expected wage increase, or reprimanded because of the quantity or quality of production. When job performance deteriorates, the patient should inform an immediate superior at work of the diagnosis. Without this information, supervisors may interpret the poor performance as due to drugs, alcohol, or irresponsibility and begin procedures for job termination. If the patient is fired, he will not be eligible for disability payments from the company. If the employer realizes that an illness is present, he is almost always supportive in obtaining retirement with disability and can occasionally provide easier work so that the patient can continue a little longer.

The second step the physician needs to take to assure that the patient receives appropriate disability benefits is to complete the Social Security Disability Determination Form adequately. Huntington's disease does not conform to any of the specific disorders for which guidelines are provided to the SSDI claims officers (U.S. DHHS 1986). Signs and symptoms relevant to HD are scattered in several different sections of the manual. Often, the HD patient does not have enough signs to qualify for disability under any one of these categories even though he cannot work. For this reason, the physician's claim that the patient is disabled needs to be supported by specific examples of task failures at work. This information can sometimes be obtained from the patient but is more fully available from the patient's supervisor at work. As discussed in chapter 3, IQ tests do not adequately reflect the patient's cognitive impairment and can be used by the disability officer as evidence that the patient is not disabled. If IQ test scores are requested, an explanation should accompany the report stating that when continually prompted, as in an IQ test, the patient can still perform above the defective range but that in a real job setting, where continual prompts are not made, the patient cannot perform. When completing the Disability Determination Form one should also keep in mind that total disability for *any* job is required for SSDI, while most private policies require only that the patient be totally disabled for his *usual* job.

Household Help

Child care services may be needed even when the patient is only mildly affected, if there are small children at home during the years of the patient's illness and if the spouse must work outside the home. This is particularly important if the patient is irritable and unpredictable in his behavior toward the children. Several clinical investigators have reported high rates of child abuse among HD families (Hughes 1924; Hans and Gilmore 1968; Dewhurst, Oliver, and McKnight 1970; Tyler et al. 1982, 1983; Pearlstein, Brill, and Mancall 1982). We have not experienced such high rates. No more than 5% of our patients have abused or seriously neglected their children, and when abuse has taken place, the guilty party has just as often been the unaffected parent as the affected parent. Patients' aggression is more often directed toward spouses.

It is probably better to arrange child care outside the home to avoid conflicts between the sitter and the patient. Low-income families who qualify for social services and medical assistance can often obtain child care or day care services through these agencies. Even a modest income, however, will disqualify families for such payments and individual arrangements must be made.

Later in the illness (anywhere from five to ten years after onset), the patient cannot be left at home alone without the risk of injury from falls or choking. Some families are forced to take this risk because of a lack of funds to hire a caregiver or, in some cases, because the patient refuses to allow outsiders in the house. Sometimes it is possible to accustom the patient gradually to a local person who can be hired for a relatively modest fee. Such a person needs to learn about the illness, what to expect, and how to respond to the patient's sometimes irascible behavior.

Communities are developing adult day care programs that can accommodate HD patients if the staff are given some education and if the patient is introduced to the setting gradually. These programs provide activity, social contacts, and supervision. The most difficult aspect is to get the patient to attend the program for the first time. It is often helpful for the physician to *order* the patient to attend day care. Usually, once the patient experiences the social opportunities associated with most such programs, he looks forward to attending.

Equipment

Late in the illness, a variety of equipment is needed for patients who are able to remain at home. Most medical insurance plans (Medicare, Medicaid, as well as private plans) cover the purchase or rental of walkers,* wheelchairs, commodes, and hospital beds. Bathroom safety equipment is not usually covered, so equipment for getting in and out of bathtubs must be purchased.

Institutional Care

HD patients often require long-term institutional care. Some become dangerously aggressive or have other intractable psychiatric symptoms. In other cases, it becomes too difficult physically for the spouse to care for the increasingly immobile patient at home, and adequate home nursing care is extremely expensive. About 28% of HD cases in Maryland are in hospitals or other institutions on any given day (unpublished data from the Maryland HD survey). A survey in the area surrounding Birmingham, England, found that at any given time about 25% of persons who are symptomatic with HD were in institutional care (Barczak et al. 1987). In the United States, three types of long-term care are available: nursing homes, chronic disease hospitals, and public psychiatric hospitals (although the latter are becoming a rare option). Veterans sometimes have the additional choice of a VA hospital. The appropriate choice depends on the physical and psychiatric characteristics of the patient. Both medical and psychiatric care can be financed by public funds if the patient has no financial assets. It is wise to recommend that the spouse consult a financial planning consultant well in advance of any expected long-term care needs.

Life-Planning Options That Can Be Made Prospectively

Several life-planning options that need to be acted upon during early adult life can decrease family burdens if the at-risk person falls ill. If families know of their risk for HD, the most prudent course is to acquire disability insurance and mortgage insurance that pay off when the holder becomes disabled. It is also helpful to work for a large company that has good disability benefits and to stay with one firm for a long time. Disability negotiations go more smoothly if the patient has long-term friends and associates at work who are willing to advocate for him during the process. Spouses of people at risk should have sufficient education to be able to earn a living if necessary. Finally, the possibility of having HD should be considered when purchasing a home. The best house for an HD patient is a one-story house. This arrangement not only is much safer but also promotes independence and allows the patient to participate in household tasks for a longer time.

---

*Be sure to order walkers that have wheels on the two front legs. HD patients lack the coordination required to lift and place ordinary walkers. The wheeled variety moves slowly forward if the patient simply leans on it.

Providing a Pleasant Environment for the Patient at Home

HD patients tend to become socially isolated and demoralized after stopping work (either in paid employment or as a homemaker). Some patients retain their capacity for initiating activities and are able to keep busy as long as they are physically able. However, many are unable to drive and may feel self-conscious in public (particularly if they have been accused falsely of drunkenness). Some are distressed that they no longer contribute to the family's functioning or feel resentful at their loss of any decision-making role. They seldom discuss these issues with their spouses and when they do, their poor judgment and quick tempers frequently turn the discussions into useless arguments.

Attention to three aspects of family life can improve the patient's self-esteem and aid in the adjustment to the limitations that HD imposes. The first involves the relationship between the patient and caregiver, usually a spouse or parent. Spouses who can learn to respond diplomatically to patients' changing feelings and capabilities and to restructure their interactions and expectations of the patient have less disrupted households. Disagreements will frequently lead to arguments, and the caregiver needs to learn to avoid confrontations and ultimatums unless the issue is quite important. It is difficult to maintain a sense of respect for patients who become unreasonable, and various strategies are needed to make the patient feel important while at the same time limiting his choices to ones that are reasonable. It is sometimes helpful to give the patient a simple choice. For example, instead of "You have to eat lunch now," suggest that the spouse try "Would you like to eat in the kitchen or the dining room?"

Second, an unvarying routine for the patient should be established. HD patients almost uniformly become attached to their routines and become anxious and resentful at any change. An appropriate routine is one that includes regular meal times, exercise, and a moderate amount of social contact. Social contacts are the most difficult aspect of the routine to maintain, partly because patients may say they do not want to socialize and partly because friends tend to fall away from anyone with a chronic illness. HD patients who have regular visits from friends look forward to them with great anticipation. The spouse should arrange regular outings with other family members, each one choosing a convenient day and time and staying with it. If necessary, the spouse can request that a good friend establish a regular visiting time. Things that occur weekly are the most pleasant for the patient, probably because they are easy to keep track of and not so frequent as to be tiring.

Obviously, changes in routine are necessary from time to time to adjust to changes in family obligations and advances in the patient's disease that make a particular activity dangerous or otherwise impossible. Changes should be made gradually. For example, if dinnertime needs to be changed, ideally it should be done gradually, a few minutes per day. Special events—family occasions, doctors' appointments, shopping for clothing—should be announced a day or two in advance followed by indirect reminders so that the patient does not forget it. Too much advance notice causes extreme anticipatory anxiety in some patients.

The third aspect of the home environment requiring attention is the physical environment, which needs to be assessed repeatedly at follow-up clinic visits. Needs change as the illness progresses, and if new needs can be anticipated, accidents may be prevented.

HD patients are prone to falls. The most common ones occur on stairs, in the bathroom, and when patients attempt to rise from chairs or sit down. The use of stairs should be minimized and all stairways provided with carpet and handrails. Bathrooms should be equipped with rubber mats, grab bars, and toilet safety rails. Sharp furniture should be removed from areas near the patient's favorite chair, thus minimizing the risk of injury in the case of a fall upon arising from the chair. Patients may resent these restrictions and attempt to continue routines and activities that have become dangerous, but the changes are usually accepted once they are in place. Homemakers may have laundry routines that can be very hard to break, such as carrying clothes baskets up and down stairs. Sometimes patients defiantly refuse to use handrails. Bathroom equipment is usually more acceptable, but walkers and wheelchairs may be resisted for a very long time. Patients are more willing to comply if "the doctor ordered it," and for this reason it is not adequate for the clinician to provide oral or written information to only the spouse. Patients are more likely to take safety suggestions seriously if the physician gives them a direct order.

The Psychological Impact of Huntington's Disease on Family Life: Changing Marital Roles

The impact of HD on the family depends on several aspects of the illness and on the nature of the household in which it occurs. These include the personality and competence of the spouse, whether the spouse was previously informed about the patient's risk for HD (Hans and Koeppen 1980), and the age at the onset of the patient's symptoms. The least troubled household is one in which the patient's symptoms begin late in life; the spouse is well informed about HD and is calm, competent, and resourceful; there have been many years of successful married life; and children are out of the home. Conversely, the most troubled family is typically one in which the patient's symptoms begin relatively early, the spouse resents not having been told about the risk for HD, the spouse is dependent or irresponsible and cannot maintain the family structure or change in response to the patient's needs, the couple has been married only a few years, and there are small children at home (Folstein, Franz et al. 1983). Even for the most prepared and competent spouse, HD provides a difficult challenge because of the change in the patient's behavior and thinking, the financial strains, the change in the marital relationship, and the risk for the children.

At first, the spouse must come to accept the diagnosis and the changes in life that it entails. Women may have to find employment for the first time and manage with less income. Men may have gradually increasing household and child care responsibilities. These tensions are worsened because they come in the context of a changing marital relationship. The affected spouse may be irritable and unreasonable or depressed and suicidal. The sexual relationship is always changed, with some patients making insistent and inappropriate sexual demands while at the same time becoming awkward in their approaches. Others become uninterested or impotent.

Spouses benefit from support and suggestions from professionals but can also be helped by other spouses who have successfully weathered similar circumstances. Concrete examples from other spouses about ways to avoid arguments, to establish routines, and to avoid the appearance of having usurped the patient's domestic and financial prerogatives are sometimes more helpful than generalities from professionals. Voluntary organizations that may have a local chapter near the family can put spouses in touch with others in similar circumstances. These organizations can not only decrease the sense of isolation felt by HD families but also provide information about local services and about current HD research.

As the disease progresses, all HD patients, even those with minimal dementia and psychiatric disturbance, become self-centered and can make unrealistic demands. The clinician's (physician's, nurse's or social worker's) office is a safe place for the patient and spouse to raise such issues. The formality of the setting inhibits serious arguments that might take place at home, and topics can be discussed and settled with the help of a professional mediator.

Spouses need to be strongly encouraged to establish regular pleasurable activities outside the household. If there is a time each day that the patient expects the spouse to be out, it becomes acceptable as part of the established routine. Many spouses feel guilty about arranging recreation that does not include the patient. However, without regular breaks the unremitting tension of caring for a chronically ill person year after year becomes unbearable.

Spouses often need help with the decision to place the patient in a nursing home or psychiatric hospital. Not only are they concerned about the possible financial burdens but also they feel it represents the ultimate abandonment and the realization of the patient's worst fears. Professionals and other spouses can be helpful in discussing these emotions and emphasizing the realities of the situation. The spouse can then be encouraged to visit several nursing homes or hospitals. Families are often prejudiced against public psychiatric hospitals, but for some patients this is much the best choice: there is more room for patients to move about, the nurses are skilled in handling abnormal behaviors, and there are always physicians on the grounds.

Once the spouse is comfortable with the decision, a discussion with the patient's sibs and children is in order. Not having the experience of caring for the patient, they may feel that the spouse should continue home care. Some relatives even take the patient into their homes rather than agreeing to institutional placement, although the arrangement is usually not successful; they soon appreciate how difficult it can be to care for some HD patients. Once family issues are resolved, the spouse may wish to discuss the best way to tell the patient about the placement plans. Some patients are relieved to enter a nursing home or hospital, particularly when they realize that someone will be constantly available to feed and dress them, to provide some social contact, and attend to any medical emergencies. Spouses experience tremendous relief after the patient is placed in a long-term care facility: it means an end to the sense of dread and tension that have come to permeate the household, a tension that may not be fully appreciated until it stops.

The Psychological Impact of Huntington's Disease on Family Life: The Effects on the Children

The effects on children of having a parent with HD vary with the children's ages and circumstances at the time of the parent's illness. If they are grown and living independently when the symptoms begin, limited evidence suggests that they are not damaged significantly psychologically (Dewhurst, Oliver, and McKnight 1970; Folstein, Franz et al. 1983). They are frequently willing to help the unaffected parent to care for the patient. If symptoms begin when the children are young and living at home, the children are at considerable psychological and social risk. The affected parent becomes inconsistent in his expectations and may be harsh in his disciplinary measures. Even if the patient remains even-tempered, he gradually becomes less able to support the children, who begin to feel responsible for the parent. Children seldom feel able to bring friends home. If the unaffected parent cannot maintain support and structure, the children are at risk (independent of their risk for HD) for developing serious behavior disturbances. Truancy, juvenile offenses, sexual promiscuity, and other behaviors reflect the failure of family support and guidance.

Occasionally, children are abused by the affected (or sometimes the unaffected) parent (Pearlstein, Brill, and Mancall 1982). It may be necessary to refer the family to social service agencies and to remove the children from the household.

All the foregoing suggestions for social and psychological management of HD patients are based on four principles. (See also Martindale and Bottomley 1980.) First, retain respect for the patient. This is difficult when patients are irritable and demanding. Their increasing handicap and dependency in every aspect of life embarrasses and demoralizes them. If treated respectfully, they retain self-respect and are more likely to respect caregivers. Second, help them to establish reasonable routines but allow them to follow their preferred routines even if they are not entirely reasonable. Third, show sympathy with their impossibly tragic situation. HD patients are amazingly stoic, given their other characteristics, about the slights of others and the limitations of their lives. They appreciate it if you let them know that you notice and are sensitive to their plight. Fourth, caregivers should protect their own health and that of any children who may be living at home. If despite adequate social and medical interventions the patient in his illness becomes a threat to the well-being of the spouse and children, then their safety, both psychological and physical, must take priority over the patient's wish to remain at home.

The Medical Management of Neurologic and Psychiatric Features

While the pharmacologic treatments for HD are palliative and do not affect the course of illness, three features of the illness can usually be helped with medication: involuntary movements, irritability, and depression. In most cases, pharmacologic interventions need to be paired with the environmental changes already discussed. Other neurologic manifestations that appear later in the illness (dysarthria, dysphagia, falls, and incontinence) can be alleviated only partially by medical and nursing surveillance.

Involuntary Movements

As discussed in chapter 2, the movement disorder in HD can be divided into two types: involuntary movements and impairment of voluntary movement. While numerous clinical trials have shown involuntary movements to respond to a variety of dopamine antagonists, voluntary movements are not usually improved and can indeed be worsened. Many patients with HD are given haloperidol at the time of diagnosis. The practice of the BHDP Research Clinic is to withhold medications for involuntary movements until they become disabling. Patients often feel more dysphoric on neuroleptics, some complain of feeling cognitively dulled, and patients treated with neuroleptics are at risk to develop tardive dyskinesia.

Modest dosages of a variety of dopamine blockers will usually improve the movements if a patient's chorea becomes severe enough to interfere with daily functioning (not all patients develop incapacitating chorea). The BHDP Research Clinic favors fluphenazine because it appears to induce less dysphoria than haloperidol and can be given as a monthly depot injection if necessary for compliance. Other experienced clinicians prefer other neuroleptics. Some patients who have excessive unwanted effects from haloperidol or fluphenazine tolerate chlorpromazine or thiothixene. The most important issue is that large dosages are not required. This opinion was recently confirmed by Barr et al. (1988), who demonstrated that no further improvement of chorea was gained at doses of haloperidol higher than 10 mg and serum concentrations between 2 and 5 mg/ml.

If chorea does not respond to neuroleptics, large doses of reserpine (9 mg per day can be administered by putting several tablets into a capsule) or other presynaptic dopamine blockers such as tetrabenazine can be tried. Reserpine precipitates depression in some patients.

Late in the course of illness the movements are less responsive to neuroleptics, probably because striatal dopamine receptors are destroyed by that time. Sometimes higher doses (e.g., 20 mg of haloperidol) will decrease the movements, but somnolence and increased choking may result. Patients with advanced disease sometimes respond transiently to one drug or another, but the chorea soon returns to its predrug levels. Fog and Pakkenberg (1980) suggested that a combination of pre- and postsynaptic dopamine blockers provides longer-lasting suppression of chorea in HD. A case report by Freinhar, Alvarez, and Chambers (1985) supported this view.

Nurses and other caregivers develop imaginative techniques for padding patients' beds and body parts to minimize the cuts and abrasions that result from constant movement.

Dysphagia

Even patients who still enjoy a reasonable quality of life are at risk for death from suffocation or pneumonia secondary to the aspiration of food. This appears to result from difficulty with coordination of the sequence of swallowing combined with unexpected inspiration of air. Late in the illness, swallowing is very labored and contributes to many deaths, directly by suffocation or aspiration or indirectly by starvation. There have not been any experimental studies to evaluate the efficacy of any of the commonly used interventions for dysphagia, but clinical experience suggests that some may be helpful.

Some patients seem to benefit from swallowing training. Leopold and Kagel (1985) outlined a program to train HD patients to chew and swallow carefully. It requires that the patient learn a rather complex procedure for eating and maintain attention to the details of the procedure right through every meal. If the patient is taught early in the illness when cognitive impairment is mild and an adequate attention span is retained, this training program seems to be helpful, even later in the course. The patient should sit upright with the neck flexed. If patients cannot do this voluntarily, a wheelchair can be equipped with straps that help maintain an upright posture. The eating sequence involves taking small bites, chewing adequately, suppressing breathing while chewing and swallowing, and searching the mouth with the tongue to be certain all food has been swallowed before taking another bite. Not all HD patients or their caregivers can follow this procedure. It is somewhat easier to maintain the routine throughout the meal if someone is feeding the patient. In this way, the rate of food intake can be controlled and oral reminders can be provided as each bite is eaten.

At the minimum, the patient's diet should be monitored and foods excluded or modified as they become difficult to swallow. Most patients swallow liquids more easily through a straw. Many need constant reminders not to eat too quickly or not to take large bites. All family members and caregivers need to be familiar with the Heimlich maneuver, and when choking becomes frequent the patient should eat only when another person is present. Swallowing is sometimes improved temporarily by low dosages of neuroleptics or a short-acting benzodiazepine before meals. The latter is particularly helpful if the patient is fearful of eating because of having experienced a severe choking episode.

Late in the illness, when swallowing becomes impossible and every meal is an ordeal, the question of gastrostomy is often raised. This difficult decision must be made by the family with input from the patient if possible. The advantage is that the patient is made more comfortable and can be adequately nourished. The disadvantage is that the patient's life can be prolonged long after he is entirely unresponsive.

Dysarthria

Speech first becomes difficult to understand, then more difficult to initiate, and if patients live a long time they become mute. Despite these difficulties with speaking, patients retain considerable understanding and have requests and information they wish to communicate. The problem has no fool-proof solution, but several methods can be used to improve communication for periods of time. When dysarthria, rather than difficulty with the initiation of speech, is the problem, the first approach is to calm the patient, reassure him that you have the time to listen, and ask him to speak very slowly. If this fails, ask him to spell the salient word; it is much easier to say individual letters clearly than whole words. Some patients can benefit from communication boards that have either the alphabet or frequently used words or phrases. The squares containing individual items must be large because patients cannot point accurately. When a patient is nearly mute but can still say yes or no, you can go through a series of likely requests and hope he indicates when you have hit on the right one.

Incontinence

All HD patients become incontinent when they are bedridden and unable to request toileting. A few, however, become incontinent of urine earlier in the course of the illness. Wheeler et al. (1985) evaluated five incontinent ambulatory HD patients urologically. Four of the five were female. Most had detrusor hyperreflexia with preserved sphincter function and apparently responded to anticholinergic medications.

Incontinence in advanced HD patients can be minimized if a pattern of urination and defecation can be discerned or established so that the patient can be taken to the toilet or a bedside commode at the appropriate times. This requires that the caregiver have the physical strength to move the patient.

Dehydration

Every summer, at least one BHDP patient is hospitalized for dehydration. HD patients for some reason are very thirsty and may drink up to three quarts of liquid per day. Most prefer caffeinated drinks, but others drink water or juices. The pathophysiologic reason for this behavior is not known, but some patients perspire excessively, especially if very choreic, and some are intolerant of hot weather.

As the illness progresses, patients may have less access to liquids because of memory trouble, choking, or decreased mobility. In hot weather or during a bout of viral gastritis they appear to be at high risk for dehydration. Jankovic (1986) reported a patient with HD who had chorea and diaphoresis and required 6 to 8 liters of fluid daily. This patient became dehydrated, with myoglobinuric renal failure, attributed to chorea-induced muscle necrosis and dehydration. Jankovic referenced similar reports of patients with other causes of dyskinesia.

Irritability

The first step in treating irritability is to decrease the complexity of the patient's environment, as previously discussed. Some patients can be helped by neuroleptic medications if environmental manipulations fail or cannot be implemented. If using fluphenazine, the initial dose should be 1 mg per day, gradually increasing up to 5 or, rarely, 10 mg per day until symptoms are controlled or unwanted effects such as excessive drowsiness, akathisia, or parkinsonism appear. An occasional patient requires less than 1 mg per day. Propranolol has also been reported to be useful for the treatment of irritability (Stewart, Mounts, and Clark 1987). A few HD patients are so irritable and aggressive that they must be chronically hospitalized to protect their families and the community. At the time of this writing, 33 of the 217 patients ascertained in the Maryland survey were hospitalized primarily for this reason.

Anxiety, Depression, and Mania

Anxiety can be treated with both environmental and pharmacologic interventions. An attempt should first be made to decrease the complexity of the patient's environment. Stopping a job that has become too difficult will usually result in a remarkable decline in anxiety. Assisting the caregiver to establish a predictable routine for the patient is also helpful. Benzodiazepines can be prescribed to be taken during times of unavoidable stress. Physicians must exercise judgment in prescribing for patients who overuse drugs unless the spouse has taken charge of medications. Most patients dislike medications and will take them only as necessary.

In the experience of most clinicians caring for HD patients, depression in HD usually responds to tricyclic antidepressants (Folstein, Folstein, and McHugh 1979), although this has not been a universal experience (Ford 1986). A therapeutic blood level is often reached at lower dosages than with non-brain-injured patients with depression, but this is unpredictable, so blood levels need to be monitored. Dosages that are too high will lead to unwanted drowsiness and failure of compliance. In the BHDP Research Clinic, the starting dose is 25 mg of nortriptyline at bedtime. Nortriptyline has less anticholinergic activity than most other tricyclics, so it less often causes dry mouth and constipation, and accurate blood levels can be obtained. Patients whose depression is unresponsive to therapeutic levels of nortriptyline may respond to the addition of lithium carbonate, which also requires monitoring of blood levels. A few patients in our experience only respond to monoamine oxidase inhibitors; a similar experience was reported by Ford (1986). There are several reports in the literature of improvement of depression with ECT (Brothers and Meadows 1955; Heathfield 1967). The Johns Hopkins psychiatric inpatient units successfully used ECT on two occasions in the last few years for patients with intractable depressive delusions who had fallen into a depressive stupor. During the Maryland survey of HD, review of patients' case notes revealed several HD patients who had been treated with ECT, usually for affective disorder that preceded any motor symptoms. The treating psychiatrist was sometimes unaware that the patient was at risk for HD.

The few studies of lithium carbonate (reviewed by Yung 1984) in HD have not taken into account whether the patients had affective disorder. At least one open trial reported improvement in involuntary movements (Mattsson 1973) although other blind trials did not. One author reported decreased irritability and aggression when lithium was given with haloperidol to patients who had high baseline ratings of those behaviors (Leonard et al. 1974). Neither drug alone had this effect, and haloperidol alone was associated with increased depression ratings. The BHDP Research Clinic staff have prescribed lithium for a number of HD patients with mania. Lithium alone has seldom alleviated or prevented recurrence of manic episodes. If these are severe and frequent enough to require pharmacologic treatment, a neuroleptic such as fluphenazine or haloperidol is usually required. Two manic patients responded to carbamazepine. Most patients' manic episodes are mild and short-lived, but occasional patients have prolonged and severe symptoms and, if they are unresponsive to treatment, must be hospitalized in a long-term care facility.

Hallucinations and Delusions

A few patients with HD have prominent hallucinations early in the course; other patients develop hallucinations and delusions late in the course. The hallucinations usually respond to neuroleptics, but larger dosages may be needed than those that control chorea and irritability. This must be titrated for each patient. Sometimes, patients have depressive symptoms along with hallucinations, and such patients usually require treatment with both tricyclic antidepressants and neuroleptics.

Experimental Treatments

Experimental Therapeutic Trials

Short-Term Trials Based on "Restoration" Paradigms   During the late 1970s, a number of drug trials were carried out based on the then-recent autopsy finding that GABA was depleted in the striatum of HD patients (e.g., Shoulson et al. 1978; Foster et al. 1983). GABA is lost because of damage to the striatal neurons that produce it. The hope was that GABA agonists would reverse the symptoms of HD as L-DOPA had done for patients with Parkinson's disease. These trials were not successful. Researchers speculated that the drugs used failed to cross the blood-brain barrier, but some of the drugs did appear to be affecting the central nervous system. Retrospectively, it can be speculated that these trials failed because the striatal neurons that make GABA also receive GABA input from other neurons, and their GABA receptors cannot be restored by increasing the available transmitter.

Trials Based on "Neurochemical Balance" Paradigms   Other trials have been based on the observation in autopsy material that dopamine is increased in the HD striatum (Sanberg and Coyle 1984). This excess, whether relative or absolute, probably results from the continued normal (or up-regulated) activity of the dopamine-producing neurons that send fibers to the striatum. At the same time, the dopamine receptors on striatal neurons are being diminished. It was reasoned that decreasing the striatal dopamine could at least partially restore the biochemical balance in the striatum and alleviate symptoms. Two general classes of dopamine antagonists have been used. Drugs such as reserpine and tetrabenazine work presynaptically on the dopamine-producing neurons or their presynaptic receptors; haloperidol, fluphenazine, and other drugs act postsynaptically on receptors on striatal neurons (e.g., Deroover et al. 1984). Both types of drugs have clearly been shown to decrease involuntary movements, particularly chorea, but have little effect on other motor abnormalities in HD such as balance, fine motor coordination, and bradykinesia. In fact, these features may be aggravated by dopamine blockers as discussed in chapter 2. Their prolonged use can cause tardive dyskinesia in HD patients.

The clinical trials of dopamine blockers have all been limited to a few weeks, but these drugs are in common use clinically for HD patients for much longer periods, up to several years. There is no indication that they can slow the course of illness or have any other long-term benefit.

A Long-Term Trial Based on a "Prevention" Paradigm   Injection of excitotoxic compounds into the striatum of rats results in neuropathologic damage that closely approximates the anatomic and biochemical changes observed in the HD striatum, as described in chapter 5. Excitotoxins are similar in structure and activity to glutamate, an amino acid thought to be an important excitatory neurotransmitter utilized by corticostriate fibers.

These findings suggested the hypothesis that HD may result from an abnormality either in the utilization or deactivation of glutamate or in the structure of its receptors that causes glutamate to act as a toxin to the striatal neurons. Under this hypothesis, damage would occur gradually as more and more striatal neurons succumbed to the effects of chronic low-grade poisoning. This led to the prediction (Shoulson et al. in press) that an effective therapeutic strategy would be to decrease the amount of available glutamate in the striatum over the long term, starting as early in the illness as possible. The outcome would be measured not in terms of symptom reversal but as a change in the rate of functional decline.

Shoulson et al. (1989) conducted a double-blind, three-year trial of baclofen, one effect of which is to decrease glutamate release. They treated HD patients whose symptoms were minimal to mild at the time of their entry into the trial. Unfortunately, baclofen did not prevent the progression of symptoms, although patients in both treatment and placebo groups progressed more slowly than expected from baseline longitudinal data on HD patients. The paradigm is still attractive, and other drugs are currently being explored that have a more specific effect on glutamate receptors.

Implants of Fetal Striatal Tissue into the Striatum in Rats

Another experimental approach to HD treatment has been to implant fetal striatal tissue into the striatum of rats that have had their striatal neurons depleted with one of the excitotoxic agents, such as kainic acid or quinolinic acid. Such implants are accepted by the brain, and the implanted neurons divide and send out branches. Systematic observations of the behavior of the implanted rats have demonstrated that some of the deficits seen after kainate treatment are reversed by the implants (Deckel et al. 1983), as are the abnormalities of drinking and feeding (Tulipan et al. 1986).

Recently, a similar procedure has been attempted in a limited number of HD patients, but the results of this experiment are not yet known.

Summary and Conclusions

The care of HD patients and their families requires a knowledge of the symptoms and course of illness and some experience and skill in helping afflicted families reorganize their lives so that they can function as the patient (or sometimes patients) changes in abilities and personal attributes. It is also helpful for the clinician to be familiar with locally available resources of care and assistance and to have some experience with medications that can alleviate some HD symptoms.

To date, therapeutic interventions based on hypothesized concepts of HD pathophysiology have been unsuccessful. However, new information is being reported daily about the structure and function of striatal neurons, fibers, and receptors which, given the current high level of research resources devoted to HD, can be readily tested for their application to HD.

10

Persons at Risk

Those who pass the fortieth year without symptoms of the disease, are seldom attacked.
—HUNTINGTON, 1872

Few empirical studies have been conducted of persons at risk for Huntington's disease. Most reports are based on small self-selected samples or are limited to anecdotal reports. One investigation of psychiatric disorder in a representative sample (Folstein, Franz et al. 1983) was based only partially on direct interviews, because of the unwillingness of many persons at risk for HD to become involved in research. Only the HD research group at the National University of Wales has succeeded in establishing an organized clinical and research relationship with most of the at-risk population in their local area (Harper et al. 1982).

The limited interest that at-risk persons have in HD research reflects in part the wish of many to avoid thinking about HD for as long as possible. However, it is likely that the paucity of investigations also stems from reticence on the part of physicians and other researchers. It is distressing to examine and test normal young adults with the realization that half of them will someday have HD.

This chapter is based largely on clinical experience with persons at risk for HD, drawing when possible upon research documentation. The experience is based on a self-selected group who have requested neurologic examination, genetic counseling, or genetic testing; on discussions with the unaffected parents of persons at risk; and on interactions with persons at risk who come to the BHDP Research Clinic in their role as caregivers to their affected parents. Altogether, about 300 at-risk persons have been formally examined at least once. Of those, only 80 wished to be formally followed longitudinally. However, information of various types is available on many more of them.

The chapter describes the characteristics of this self-selected group of persons at risk, offers suggestions for their care, and discusses the BHDP protocol for the genetic testing of persons at risk.

Case Example: Choosing to Be Tested for Huntington's Disease

Kathy Miller's mother was hospitalized in a public psychiatric hospital because of HD when Kathy was 5 years old. Her father was unable to care for her and her brother, and they lived first with their maternal grandmother and later in a series of foster homes. They were taken to visit their mother regularly, but Kathy's memories of the visits are of sitting on a hard bench in a waiting area for long periods of time, waiting for her grandmother to return. She was frightened of her mother and of the other patients in the ward.

After a tumultuous early adolescence, Kathy was finally "brought under control" by a foster family who was able to convince her of her own value as an individual and of her potential to be a happy and productive person. She knew of her risk for HD and was convinced she would be affected. Because she wanted a family, she decided to marry and have children at a young age, hoping that her family would be grown by the time she became affected. Her husband agreed to this plan, and they had four children. The marriage was a happy one, and the spouses enjoyed each other and their children, both believing that their time together would be short.

Kathy and her husband attended the BHDP Research Clinic shortly after it opened. They wanted to "register" so that they could be informed of any treatments. Kathy wished to be examined, and her neurologic examination was normal. Her husband telephoned occasionally to voice his concerns that Kathy was forgetting things and occasionally appeared to be anxious. He was convinced that these behaviors indicated HD but never shared his fears with her. They had four young children and Kathy held a part-time job at the time. Yearly examinations continued to be normal but, because of her husband's reports, the examining physician considered Kathy to be "at risk, suspicious."

As soon as presymptomatic testing became available, Kathy brought her brother, by now clearly affected with HD, to the clinic for documentation of his diagnosis and to obtain a blood sample to be used for testing Kathy. The results of Kathy's screening neurological examination for the testing program were again normal. She was, therefore, accepted for the program but given small hope of an informative test because only she, her brother, and her unaffected father were available for testing.

In several sessions with a psychologist, Kathy and her husband, who served as her confidant even though she had to convince him that testing was a good idea, discussed their wish for testing and its possible consequences on their lives. Kathy's main purpose for wanting testing was to protect her children should she become affected. She did not want them to have to experience her illness, and in the event she had HD she intended to implement a plan for her own care away from home. She also had thought of a way for her husband to obtain help in caring for their children. Her husband agreed that this plan was reasonable, but feared the outcome of the test. Kathy had her blood drawn and took the cognitive, personality, and other tests that were part of the research protocol, and waited for her results. She was told that when the laboratory had completed the study, they would telephone and give her the information either that the test was uninformative or that there was a result. In the latter case, she could then make an appointment to come to the hospital with her husband if she wished the result to be disclosed.

Remarkably, she and her brother were both heterozygous for the markers, and each of them had different markers (see figure app5.5 for her family as an example of an informative family). Therefore, she could be told that her risk for having HD was less than 1%. She was telephoned and told that the laboratory had a result, and an appointment for disclosure was arranged for the next week. An earlier appointment was suggested, but her husband could not arrange to be away from work until a week later.

During that week Kathy and her husband alternated between optimism and near panic, sure that the outcome would be bad. They discussed whether they should call it off, but Kathy was determined that, whatever the outcome, she needed to know it for the benefit of their children. For the two nights before disclosure they slept little. Immediately upon their arrival at the hospital, they were ushered into the counseling room and told that Kathy's risk for HD was less than 1%. Kathy screamed and cried and kissed everyone. Her husband didn't believe it at first and sat silent until it sank in, and then he also cried.

Characteristics of Persons at Risk for Huntington's Disease
Personal Features

Persons at risk for HD are in most ways ordinary people. Some are careful; some take risks. Some are optimistic; others fear the worst. Some are hard working; some are not. They have the average range of interests, skills, and talents. An individual's personal traits appear to bear little relationship to whether he has the HD gene or not. This is not to deny that personal traits may change in a somewhat stereotyped way as the illness begins (as described in earlier chapters), but while they are well, persons with the gene are not reliably distinguishable from their sibs who are without it.

The first 147 at-risk persons who volunteered for the BHDP research project were asked to complete the Eysenck Personality Inventory, which rates two personality traits along a continuum: introversion/extraversion and neuroti-cism/nonneuroticism. The distribution of these traits in the at-risk persons did not differ from the distribution in the general population (table 10.1). However, persons who later became affected (and were diagnosed as having HD an average of 3 years later) were more likely to have high scores of neuroticism. Similarly, most persons at risk score in the normal range on the General Health Questionnaire, a self-rated questionnaire assessing mood and anxiety, but those who became affected soon after indicated more dysphoria.

Table 10.1. Personality Traits and Mood in Persons at Risk When Tested

Test	Total Population	Still Normal	Now Suspicious or Affected	P[a]
EPI	N = 147	N = 106	N = 41	
EXT/INT ($\bar{X}$)	11.4	11.4	11.6	NS
NEU/NONNEU ($\bar{X}$)	8.2	7.5	10.0	.016
LIE Score ($\bar{X}$)	3.3	3.3	3.1	NS
GHQ	N = 161	N = 113	N = 48	
% Abnormal	20%	16%	31%	.03
Depression	N = 316	N = 244	N = 72	
% with DX	9%	4.5%	25%	.000
QNE	N = 307	N = 236	N = 71	
Mean score	2.91	2.56	4.06	.004

[a]P values are for comparisons of the still normal group with the now suspicious or affected group.
Note: 307 self-selected persons at 50% risk for HD were examined neurologically using the Quantified Neurologic Examination (QNE) and classified as unaffected; 147 completed the Eysenck Personality Inventory (EPI) which rates extraversion/introversion (EXT/INT), neuroticism/ nonneuroticism (NEU/NONNEU) and lying, a measure of denial of unfavorable traits; 161 completed the 30-item General Health Questionnaire (GHQ). The distribution of scores for all tests were in the normal range. Persons who became affected or questionably affected within 3 to 5 years had higher initial scores for neuroticism on the EPI, were more likely to score in the abnormal range on the GHQ (5 or more), were more likely to have had an episode of depression, and scored more points on the QNE.

These clinical observations may be somewhat surprising in light of the incredible burdens borne by persons who know that they are at 50% risk for a fearful illness. Many grow up in a household where one parent was chronically ill, cognitively and emotionally disordered, and often difficult to manage. Others are burdened during adult life by caring for an affected parent. All those who are aware of their risk are burdened by the nagging fear that HD may hit them at any time, and half have the additional burden of the HD gene, which may exert its effects long before clinical diagnosis is possible.

Not everyone bears these burdens with equal ease, but it is surprising how many at-risk persons seem to enjoy life and accomplish to their levels of ability despite their burdens. When asked how much they think about HD, most at-risk persons who are not actively caring for an affected relative say that thoughts of HD occur either infrequently or that they think about it when they trip, drop something, or forget something. For the most part they are able to replace thoughts of HD easily. They say that occasionally they have a day or even a week during which they think often about HD and what would happen to them and their families if they became affected. During these periods, they may seek comfort and reassurance from their spouses or friends. Reassurance is often sought in the context of a joke after tripping or dropping something. Many say that the subject is too painful for both them and their families to allow many serious discussions.

At-risk persons (usually women) who are caring for an affected parent think about HD considerably more because of its constant presence in their lives. These people often appear sad and are easily brought to tears. They are also tired, like all HD caregivers. The few who have chosen to have presymptomatic testing at Johns Hopkins have been unaffected, and that has helped improve their frame of mind.

A few individuals known to the BHDP have been preoccupied by constant thoughts and fears about HD. These persons appear to have been predisposed to their reactions by certain personal traits, particularly obsessionality or hypochondriasis. Some of these individuals have the HD gene, and others do not.

These observations apply to persons who have known about HD and their risk for a long time, sometimes since childhood. When people first learn about their risk for HD, especially when they are adults at the time the information is disclosed, they are completely preoccupied with thoughts of it for a while. Children and teenagers are often less upset, children because they cannot entirely appreciate the implications for themselves, and teenagers because of the wonderful sense of optimism and invulnerability characteristic of most late adolescents and young adults. To them, sickness and death seem a long way off.

The reaction of an adult who first learns of his risk for HD is not unlike grief mixed with anger. There is first a sense of disbelief, panic, and shock. This gives way to feelings of helplessness and powerlessness to undo fate, accompanied by a strong feeling of anger toward the parents. The at-risk person is angry with the affected parent for having put him at risk, especially if the parent was aware of HD at the time the children were conceived. He may also be angry with the unaffected parent for not disclosing the information sooner (or at all, if the information was obtained from someone else). These and similar thoughts are completely preoccupying for a time and then subside somewhat, returning in waves with the recurrence of the associated emotions.

Eventually, most people come to terms with their risk for HD. They become able to stop thinking about it most of the time, although the fear is always under the surface. Some people are unable to think about it or discuss it with their families for several years after learning about it, and others are never able to tolerate the subject. Others deal with the fear by taking whatever precautions they can, such as obtaining a secure job and disability insurance. Still others attack their fear actively by becoming involved in research or fund-raising. Occasionally, persons claim to be genuinely unconcerned.

Most people at risk hide their burden from all but their family members and one or two friends. Rarely do they tell their employers that they are at risk. Unless and until they begin to have symptoms of HD, they are known to their friends and in their communities as ordinary people.

Psychiatric Features

In an attempt to assess the rate, type, and correlates of psychiatric disorder in adolescents and young adults at risk for HD, Folstein, Franz et al. (1983) selected 34 HD patients who were parents of children 15 years old and older. Consecutive HD patients who met these criteria were drawn from a roster of patients ascertained during the Maryland HD survey. Thus the parents were not selected for having children who would necessarily be cooperative with the study. This limited the quality of information that could be obtained about their offspring but made it possible to investigate the psychiatric disorders of a representative group of offspring of HD parents. When possible, the offspring were directly interviewed. Otherwise, information was obtained about them from as many sources as possible, usually one or more siblings and the unaffected parent.

The psychiatric disorders found in the 112 offspring are summarized in table 10.2. The most commonly diagnosed condition was adolescent conduct disorder and its adult equivalent, antisocial personality disorder. These diagnoses were correlated with the experience of a disorganized household, an experience usually related to having an *affected* parent with an early onset of symptoms and an *unaffected* parent who was unable to maintain a stable family environment. The disorders of conduct often subsided when the child left the household. These findings are in agreement with those of Dewhurst (1970), who described a single large at-risk sibship in which the presence of antisocial behavior during adolescence was unrelated to the eventual development of HD.

The second most common disorder diagnosed in the offspring was major affective disorder. This diagnosis did not correlate with the early family experience, but was found more often in offspring who were eventually diagnosed as having HD and correlated with having an affected parent with affective disorder.

Mild anxiety disorders are also found among the offspring of HD patients. The antecedents and correlates of this condition are not known, but the causes

Table 10.2. Psychiatric Disorder among Adolescent and Adult Offspring of Persons with Huntington's Disease

Disorder	Males	Females	Total
Conduct disorder or antisocial personality	18	10	28 (25%)
Major affective disorder	9	11	20 (18%)
Other	1	8	18 (16%)
No disorder	25	29	54 (48%)
Any disorder	33	25	58 (52%)
	(N = 58)	(N = 54)	(N = 112)

are likely to be mixed. In our experience, some persons are made anxious by the stress of being at risk for HD. On the other hand, anxiety is also an early manifestation of HD itself.

While the rate of psychiatric disorder was high, most conditions (anxiety and depression) were mild or had been present during adolescence (conduct disorder). A few people had antisocial criminal behavior that continued into adulthood. Very few of these at-risk persons had sought treatment for their symptoms.

Cognitive Features

There may be small group differences in cognition between at-risk persons who later develop HD and those who are free of the gene. Reed et al. (1958) reported that persons who later became affected achieved lower employment status than did their unaffected siblings. However, the data did not allow a comparison of the job status of the two groups at similar ages, so the unaffected sibs may simply have had a longer time to progress in their jobs.

Lyle and Gottesman (1979) followed a group of 88 at-risk persons in Minnesota who had had cognitive testing 15 to 20 years earlier (the Bender Gestalt test, the Shipley-Hartford Retreat scale, and the Wechsler intelligence scales). The initial scores on the tests were lower for the subjects who had HD by the time of follow-up than for those subjects still without symptoms at follow-up. However, there was a wide variation in the scores within both groups of subjects, and none of the scores alone or in any combination could be used to predict with more than 78% accuracy which individuals would develop HD.

Strauss and Brandt (1986) noted that HD patients had a distinct pattern of scores on the subtests of the WAIS, as described in chapter 3. They therefore assessed the WAIS subtest pattern of 38 at-risk persons to see whether any of them had the same pattern as HD patients. Seventeen had WAIS patterns similar (though higher in absolute level) to those of HD patients and 21 had profiles similar to those of normals. No clinical differences could be found between the subgroups, but longer-term follow-up, or the results of genetic linkage analysis, would be required either to confirm or to refute this attempted classification.

Despite small group differences, it is clear that presymptomatic HD heterozygotes are extremely variable in their cognitive functioning, ranging from persons with advanced degrees to unskilled laborers, and as a group are not cognitively impaired by any criteria before the onset of illness.

Neurologic Features

Neurologic examinations of at-risk persons who are free of the HD gene are normal, despite their anxiety at being examined. In the BHDP population (table 10.1), those at-risk persons who remained normal 5 years after examination, scored well below a conservative cut-off of seven points on the QNE. (This cut-off was established by examining normal individuals not at risk for HD; none scored above five points). On the other hand, neurologic examinations of presymptomatic adults who are known to have the HD gene may be either normal or slightly abnormal. Asymptomatic heterozygotes often have minor abnormalities of eye movements, slight slowing or dysrhythmia when performing rapid alternating hand movements (dysdiadochokinesis), or very slight involuntary movements of the fingers when the arms are held forward at 90° and the eyes closed. Young et al. (1988) have formally demonstrated this. These investigators carried out genetic testing on 21 at-risk persons that they had classified as unaffected. The 11 subjects with normal genetic markers had neurologic examinations that were entirely normal. Of the 10 at-risk persons with the HD marker, 7 had minor abnormalities on a quantified clinical neurologic examination (Young et al. 1988). This result provides convincing validation for the use of a low diagnostic threshold in persons who are known to be at 50% risk and have minor neurologic signs.

The interpretation of a neurologic examination of an adult who is at 50% risk and whose genotype is unknown can be difficult. Those with an absolutely normal examination (no points at all on the Quantified Neurologic Examination) may still develop HD at some time in the future. On the other hand, even minor neurologic signs, which might not be of significance in someone drawn from the general population, should not be ignored in someone at 50% risk for HD. While such signs should not be used in isolation for diagnosis, they suggest a possible neurologic abnormality, and the individual should be reexamined regularly if he wishes to know whether he has HD. Caution in the interpretation of minor signs is important. Two persons in the BHDP testing program who were later revealed by genetic testing to have only a 1% chance for having the HD gene, had slight signs on neurologic examination. A similar experience was reported by Koroshetz et al. (1988).

The Care of Persons at Risk for Huntington's Disease

The care of persons at risk for HD takes place in several different contexts. Unaffected parents often request advice about explaining HD to their at-risk children, including the best way to inform them about their risk for HD. Occasionally, persons at risk seek care because of their emotional symptoms, and some persons at risk, particularly those who find out about HD only during adult life, request genetic counseling.

Telling Children about Their Being at Risk

It is extremely painful for parents of children at 50% risk for HD to inform their children of that risk. Usually the unaffected parent takes responsibility for disclosing the information; the affected parent will seldom do it. Tyler and Harper (1983) asked parents whether they thought that their children should be informed, and most unaffected parents (74%) agreed that they should be. However, only 37% of them had actually informed their children. Our clinical experience suggests that parents' reticence stems mainly from their natural wish to protect their children from pain and harm. Usually parents intend to tell their children but keep putting it off. Some parents (and this is not rare) make an active decision to hide the hereditary nature of HD from their children and from everyone else. The reasons for this decision are that the parents may believe that HD is shameful or may fear that their children will be unmarriageable if they disclose their risk to prospective mates or if the information is circulated in the community.

Our experience suggests that parents should be strongly encouraged to tell their children about their risk for HD during adolescence, between ages 14 and 16, depending on the child's maturity. Before this time the children have trouble comprehending the information, and if they understand it at all may believe that they will *definitely* get HD, and probably soon. Adolescents are old enough to comprehend that they are not affected but at risk, and are beginning to make their own decisions about their future for which the information is important. They often have figured out themselves that they are at risk through knowing affected relatives and gaining information from television programs. An adolescent occasionally calls the BHDP social worker to discuss his risk because his parents have not brought it up and he wishes to spare the parents' feelings.

Parents can be reassured that the information may not be as painful for their children to receive as it is for them to give. Parents should also be cautioned that the failure to provide the information could damage their relationship with their children and their children's relationship with any future spouse. When adolescents find out about their risk from others, they may interpret the parents' failure to inform them as a betrayal, a withholding of information that they need for full self-knowledge and planning for the future. If the child goes on to marry and is unable (or unwilling) to tell his spouse about his risk for HD, there can be serious problems with trust in the marriage (Hans and Koeppen 1980). The spouse is never sure who was responsible for the deception. The fear of unmarriageability is largely unfounded, anyway. Most prospective spouses are willing to go ahead in spite of the knowledge, and often adopt a protective attitude toward their at-risk mate. An individual who is not willing to go forward with the marriage after hearing about the risk for HD may not be the best person for an at-risk person to marry. As discussed in earlier chapters, spouses of HD patients bear tremendous burdens, and not every spouse is willing to bear them.

Psychotherapy for Persons at Risk

In part, persons at risk consult psychotherapists for the same things that other people do. Marital problems, anxiety, depression, and alcoholism are the most common reasons for seeking consultation. Among the at-risk persons consulting a psychotherapist, some will have symptoms that probably result from having the HD gene. This is particularly true of anxiety and depression, and psychotherapists seeing at-risk persons should keep this in mind and, unless there are important reasons not to, should discuss with the patient the possible relationship between HD and these symptoms. If the depression is severe, such discussions should be delayed, although the spouse should be informed. If there are slight involuntary movements or increasing apathy, a neurologic consultation should be obtained. Again, circumstances vary, and the patient's best interest should be served.

A few persons at risk consult a psychotherapist because of overwhelming fears about HD. Most at-risk persons come to terms with their fears and learn to minimize the effect of HD on their lives, but some become preoccupied with searching for HD symptoms in themselves. Although all persons at risk do this to a certain extent, only a few repeatedly consult physicians despite reassurances that their examinations are normal. When reassurance has clearly failed, they will usually be referred to a psychiatrist or other therapist. The treatment plan should be tailored to the individual circumstances but should always involve an exploration of the patients' experience with HD and the meaning of the risk in their lives.

Genetic Counseling for Huntington's Disease

At-risk persons who request genetic counseling represent a small portion of the at-risk population and, like other people seeking information about genetics, are better educated than the general population.

The process of genetic counseling for persons at risk for HD includes several steps. First, the counselor should be clear about what questions are being asked. Persons at risk for HD usually request two general types of information; the risk for HD to themselves, and the risk for HD to children they now have or may yet have. Other issues may also be on their mind, including educational and job choices and the purchase of housing or insurance. Some at-risk persons may wish to know only what HD is but not whether they have it themselves, or they may wish advice about how to care for an affected family member. Some persons at risk for HD have to overcome considerable internal resistance to seeking genetic counseling, and they can be frightened off if more information is provided than they are prepared to hear.

Second, the counselor should be sure that the diagnosis is correct. This can be accomplished by taking a family history and obtaining a description of the clinical features of persons reported to be affected with HD, followed by an examination (preferably) or review of the medical records and any autopsy reports of the affected parent. Chapter 8 includes detailed suggestions for diagnostic evaluation.

Third, the at-risk person should be examined *if appropriate*. Some persons requesting genetic counseling are already affected. Others have minor neurologic or psychiatric abnormalities that probably imply a high risk for HD, so an accurate estimate of risk cannot be established without a neurologic and psychiatric examination. A neurologic examination is extremely frightening for many at-risk persons and should not be carried out without their consent. Many at-risk persons come to the BHDP Research Clinic *only* for the purpose of gathering information and do not wish to be examined. Persons who decline to be examined need to realize that the risk estimate given presumes that their neurologic examination is normal.

Fourth, the information requested should be provided. Because the age at onset of HD is influenced by the age at onset and sex of the affected parent as well as the age of the person requesting counseling, these should be taken into account if the at-risk person requests a numerical estimate of risk (see figure app5.1). Very few persons requesting genetic counseling for HD have a negligible risk for HD unless they are quite elderly, and they should be reminded that even persons with low risks and normal examinations can develop symptoms in the future.

It is important for the clinician to provide the information in a supportive but neutral fashion. It is not the role of any professional providing genetic counseling to prescribe a plan for behavior. For example, some at-risk persons request an opinion about childbearing. They may ask, "Do you think we should have children?" or "What would you do if you were at risk?" These questions should be reframed to allow the couple to consider their options for action and the consequences of those actions, so that they make their own decisions. The purpose of genetic counseling is not to give such advice, which can be resented as intrusive even if it is requested. Whether to have children is a personal decision, and the only role of a genetic counselor is to provide the most accurate information possible about the counselee's risk for HD, the risk to any children, and the burden of the illness if the counselee does not already know it.

Some suggestions can appropriately be made about other issues. For example, the person at risk should be informed that genetic testing for HD is possible under some circumstances and that it is wise to store blood from affected relatives in case he or other family members later decide to have testing. At-risk persons should be reminded that, should they later become affected, a one-story house will be safer and prolong independence. They should be advised to consider insurance and disability benefits when choosing employment, and to seek advice about what type of life insurance is appropriate for them.

Genetic Testing for Huntington's Disease

As described in chapter 7, Gusella et al. (1983) discovered a genetic marker (G8) at the tip of chromosome 4 that is linked to (located near) the HD gene. The ultimate goal is to find the HD gene itself. The knowledge of the gene's approximate location makes it possible for clinicians to provide very accurate information (with only a 1% error rate) about the risk for HD to at least some persons. As will be explained below, having a marker (but not the gene itself) means that the DNA of several family members must be examined to estimate the risk for HD to an asymptomatic individual. If sufficient family members are not available, the at-risk person cannot be given any information (Harper and Sarfarazi 1985; Maestri et al. 1987). Once the HD gene itself is discovered, it will be only a short time until the exact mutation (or mutations if there are different mutations in different families) is known. At that time, it will be possible to test any individual for HD—without the need for information about any other family members—with very high accuracy. The discovery of the gene is probably not far off, but the test, as it is currently performed using linkage analysis, is explained in appendix 5.

The Johns Hopkins Protocol for Genetic Testing for Huntington's Disease

At Johns Hopkins, presymptomatic genetic testing for HD is being carried out according to a research protocol approved by the Johns Hopkins Committee on Clinical Investigation. The protocol is similar to those in current use at other universities offering testing. Several meetings were held among the groups planning to start testing to discuss the protocols, particularly the ethical aspects of testing. The decision to begin testing under experimental protocols was based on concerns for the well-being of the at-risk persons choosing to be tested. Never before in human history had a person been able to choose to know, with a high degree of probability, that sometime in the future he would die of a fatal, inherited disease. How people would respond to this information was unknown. There was a serious possibility that significant psychiatric and social problems would result from this knowledge. There is no treatment for HD at the present time, and depression is common among presymptomatic heterozygotes.

It seemed important to evaluate the effects of testing in a systematic way. The evaluation was designed to answer questions about several unknown aspects of testing. How many people would be interested in having testing? Could testing be done safely, and if so, what safeguards would be needed to protect those choosing to be tested? Of those requesting testing, which ones might be at particular risk for psychological or social difficulties after testing? How should a presymptomatic testing program be designed, and how much would testing cost?

Without having answers to any of these questions at the beginning of the testing program, the initial BHDP protocol was designed to provide maximal protection for those persons who requested testing. First, the Baltimore center initially offered presymptomatic genetic testing to only at-risk persons living within 150 miles of Baltimore. The purpose of this geographical restriction was to ensure that persons being told that they were likely to have the HD gene had ready access to the center's professional staff for support and care. Because no serious consequences of testing have yet occurred, we now offer testing to persons in all states bordering Maryland. Second, each person requesting testing is required to have a confidant, a close friend or family member, who attends some of the pretest counseling sessions and who receives the test results along with the at-risk person. Third, testing is not offered to anyone whose ability to give informed consent for testing is compromised in any way. For this reason, persons who are mentally retarded, who have psychotic symptoms, or who are depressed at the time they are examined are not offered testing. Persons who are depressed may reapply after successful treatment for the depression. Anyone under pressure from family members to have testing is also considered to be unable to give informed consent. If there is evidence that an at-risk person is being pressured into testing, the issue is discussed in pretest counseling before any decision about proceeding is made. Finally, the Johns Hopkins testing program accepts only adults or adolescent minors who are independent of their parents. The decision to know one's future health was, in our judgment, one that should be made by only the person himself. Testing children would put this decision in the hands of their parents.

Objections can be raised to each of these principles on the grounds that the protocol is overly paternalistic and limits the person's right to privacy. If experience provides convincing evidence that not all these precautions are necessary (as it has with the geographical restriction), they may be reconsidered. Our primary goal is to do no harm.

The testing protocol in current use at Johns Hopkins is explained below. While it would no longer be necessary to confirm the diagnosis in other family members or to obtain blood samples from multiple relatives if a specific gene based test were available, most of the counseling and follow-up aspects of testing would remain unchanged. The psychological test battery will probably be considerably shortened after enough people have been through the protocol to determine which tests are useful in predicting the need for posttest surveillance.

The Documentation of Adequate Family Structure   The first step in the genetic testing protocol is to ascertain whether a sufficient number of family members are available to provide a potentially informative test. Some examples of families that have an informative family structure and others with an uninformative structure are given in appendix 5. Families with an informative structure are only *potentially* informative. Whether they will actually be informative depends upon the pattern of marker polymorphisms among the relatives. Currently, so many markers are available for use (Gusella et al. 1983; Gilliam et al. 1987; Wasmuth et al. 1988) that most tests are informative.

Neurologic Examination of the Person Requesting Testing   Next, the person at risk requesting testing (referred to hereafter as the ARRT) is examined neurologically. The Johns Hopkins testing program accepts for testing only those persons who are clinically unaffected with HD. There are three reasons for this decision. First, the test can be uninformative, and if an individual has clear clinical features of HD and is requesting a diagnosis, it seems unreasonable to withhold diagnosis on the basis of an uninformative genetic test. Second, until recently the accuracy of a diagnosis based on the test (95%) was probably less than that of a diagnosis based on clear clinical features of HD in a person with well-documented HD in the family. Third, the Johns Hopkins testing program is based on a research protocol designed to assess how asymptomatic individuals react to presymptomatic testing. The use of the test for diagnostic confirmation will be discussed below.

Psychiatric Examination of the Person Requesting Testing   At the visit for the neurologic examination, the ARRT is interviewed by a nurse using the Schedule for Affective Disorder and Schizophrenia, Lifetime Version (SADS-L). This structured psychiatric interview also covers other psychiatric disorders, such as anxiety, drug and alcohol abuse, panic disorder, phobias, and antisocial personality disorder. If a major psychiatric illness is suspected, based on either the SADS-L or other evidence from the interview or history, a psychiatrist examines the individual before proceeding further with the protocol. If major affective disorder is present, the decision to accept the ARRT into the testing protocol is deferred pending treatment. To date, no one has had schizophrenic symptoms. Other disorders have not been used to exclude persons from testing.

The Diagnosis of Family Members   Once the ARRT has been accepted for testing, the next step is to document that the affected family members whose blood samples are required for testing actually have HD and that the elderly at-risk persons to be used as "escapees" are in fact clinically unaffected. All relatives being used in the test as escapees should be examined by a physician experienced with HD to be certain that they are free of signs of the illness. Affected members should also be examined or, if that is not possible, their medical records should be reviewed.

Psychological Testing   Detailed psychological testing is conducted over two or more sessions. The purpose of such testing is threefold: (1) to determine whether any psychological variables (especially cognitive deficits) are associated with having the marker which may be useful for prediction in and of themselves; (2) to establish a baseline from which to measure any psychological morbidity attributable to the disclosure of test results; and (3) to determine whether constellations of personality and emotional traits, cognitive characteristics, and social variables can predict the ARRT's response to receiving genetic test results.

Pretest Counseling   At the same time the relatives are being screened, the ARRT begins pretest counseling. He attends several 90-minute counseling sessions with one of the two psychologists on the presymptomatic testing staff. The ARRT's confidant is required to attend some of these sessions, and other family members may also be included. There are several purposes of counseling. One is to explain the nature of a test based on genetic linkage analysis and to ascertain that the test and its limitations are understood. Another is to discuss with the individual his motivations for requesting testing, especially to be sure he has considered all the possible consequences of testing, and to bring to his attention possible consequences (particularly unhappy ones) that he may not have considered. The counseling sessions also allow the staff and the ARRT to become well acquainted with each other and to form a trusting relationship. This relationship makes it more likely that the ARRT will honestly divulge any pressure being placed on him to have testing and will discuss other hidden agenda. Most important, the relationship should make it more likely that, in the event of a bad test outcome, the tested person will request any needed help and support from the staff.

During the pretest counseling period, the at-risk person meets the social worker or psychiatrist who will be available for psychotherapy and other support after testing.

Disclosure of the Test Results   Once the counselor and the ARRT agree that all the issues have been adequately discussed and the ARRT decides that he wishes to proceed with testing, the laboratory begins to analyze the DNA samples. The ARRT and his advocate are told that they will be contacted when there is a result. If the test is uninformative, blood from other family members may be requested. If the test remains uninformative, the ARRT is telephoned with this information.

If the test is informative, the ARRT is told that there is a result, asked if he still wants the information, and if he does, a disclosure session is scheduled. Throughout the process, the person requesting testing and his confidant are reminded that the testing process can be stopped at any time up until the test results have actually been disclosed.

If the test shows that the individual is highly likely to have the HD gene, appropriate support is given as needed, and he is telephoned the day following disclosure and frequently thereafter for the first two weeks.

Clinical Follow-up   Clinical follow-up is offered free of charge as part of the Johns Hopkins testing program. Other programs have not offered this service but have required that the ARRT have a designated therapist before entering the protocol. In the Johns Hopkins program, each person tested, regardless of the test outcome, is assigned to either a social worker or a psychiatrist for clinical follow-up. The tested individual may choose to keep in contact with the therapist by telephone, to schedule an unlimited number of visits, or not to contact the therapist at all except for visits during scheduled research follow-up sessions (see below). The purpose of having two different kinds of professionals as therapists is to assess the usefulness of each set of skills to the tested individuals.

Research Follow-up   During the first year after testing, the tested individuals are reevaluated every 3 months and in subsequent years, every 6 months. Follow-up visits include a neurologic examination, an abbreviated form of the SADS (SADS-Change), measures of social supports and psychological well-being, cognitive testing, and an unstructured interview with the therapist and the psychologist who did the pretest counseling.

The Outcome of Presymptomatic Testing

Not many eligible at-risk persons have requested testing. Of 387 persons who were sent letters announcing its availability only 89 requested testing. These 89 persons are better educated than our clinic-based at-risk sample as is typical of persons requesting genetic counseling. There were an equal number of men and women with a mean age of about 35 years. Those who had positive tests (see below) were somewhat younger. Thirteen were not accepted for testing (3 because of depression and 10 because they had neurologic signs of HD at the time of their initial neurologic examination). Of the 53 persons who had completed testing by 15 September 1988, 9 had positive tests (95–99% likely to have HD) and 29 had negative tests (95–99% likely not to have HD). Possible reasons for this distribution are the age distribution of the sample and our rigorous screening of persons who had mild neurologic manifestations and depression. Fifteen have had tests that are, so far, uninformative; DNA from additional family members will decrease this number.

None of the nine persons with positive tests had any serious psychiatric or social sequelae to date, but some have had the information for only a short time. Of the three who had the test information for more than a year, one person had a minor depression and increased irritability, and one lost a job. There have been no divorces or other social consequences. Meissen et al. (1988) reported similar findings. Nearly all remain convinced that testing was the right thing for them. Of the 28 with negative tests, one woman became pregnant and gave birth, and one woman separated from her husband and children.

There were some differences in baseline (before the disclosure of test results) neuropsychological test performances in those persons who tested positive and those who tested negative (figure 10.1). Both groups had experienced the same

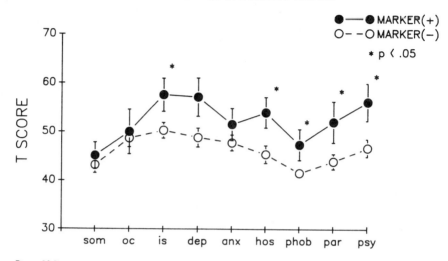

Figure 10.1. SCL-90 Overall Baseline profile. *som* = somatization; *oc* = obsessive-compulsive; *is* = interpersonal sensitivity; *dep* = depression; *anx* = anxiety; *hos* = hostility; *phob* = phobic anxiety; *par* = paranoid ideation; *psy* = psychoticism.

number of adverse life events as measured by a modified version of Dohrenwend's Life Events scale (Dohrenwend et al. 1982). However, those who subsequently tested positive reported having experienced significantly more distress (p < .05) from these life events than persons who tested negative. Scores on a psychological symptom checklist, SCL-90R (Derogotis 1983), were higher at baseline in test-positive persons but did not increase after the disclosure of test results. The SCL-90R scores of those who tested negative decreased even further after testing (Figure 10.2) (Brandt et al. 1988).

These findings are consistent with our clinical experience that some individuals become more emotionally labile as disease onset nears. The test results underscore the importance of monitoring individuals who test positive. These test-positive persons are vulnerable psychologically and will become more so with time.

The cost of testing is substantial. Counseling costs about $1000 and the average cost of DNA analysis and genetic risk estimation is $3000. The latter cost will decrease substantially when testing is based on known mutations instead of linkage analysis.

Using Genetic Testing to Confirm the Diagnosis of Huntington's Disease

It is sometimes possible to use the genetic test to confirm the diagnosis in persons who already have clinical features of HD or who have mild neurologic

SCL–90 R: GLOBAL SEVERITY INDEX

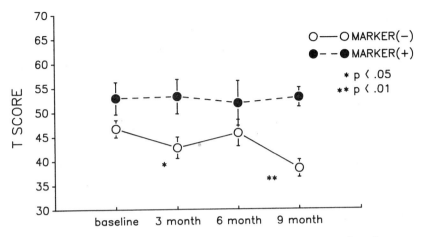

Figure 10.2. SCL-90 R: Global Severity Index. Persons in the presymptomatic testing program completed the Symptom Checklist 90, Revised (SCL-90R) before testing (baseline) and at each three-month follow-up visit. Before knowing the results of testing, those persons who later tested positive had higher SCL-90 scores than those who tested negative on five scales. At follow-up, scores for the test positive persons remained stable, while the test negative persons admitted to progressively fewer symptoms. Scores of all subjects (who had been prescreened for psychiatric disorder) were well within the normal range.

signs that are difficult to interpret. The markers now available provide information that is 99% accurate, and if the family structure is informative, more than 90% of the tests are informative. However, other affected and unaffected family members are required, just as with presymptomatic testing. The test is not at all useful in the most common occasion of uncertain diagnosis, when the family history is apparently negative. Genetic testing for HD in this circumstance will require a test based on the known mutation(s) in the HD gene itself.

On one occasion, the BHDP used genetic linkage analysis to confirm that a family with unusual clinical and neuropathologic features had a mutation at the HD locus (Zweig et al. in press). However, this requires a fairly large kindred.

Using Genetic Testing for Prenatal Diagnosis

It is possible to use genetic testing for prenatal diagnosis. This can be done in two ways: disclosure testing and nondisclosure testing. Disclosure testing applies when one of the parents has HD or has had a positive test for HD. The requirements for family structure are the same as those for presymptomatic testing, and the possible test outcomes will be *uninformative*, *positive*, or *negative*, with these words having probabilistic meanings as explained above.

Nondisclosure testing can be carried out for fetuses of at-risk persons who do not have enough family members to provide more accurate information or for fetuses of at-risk persons who choose not to have presymptomatic testing but who wish to avoid transmitting the affected gene to their children. In nondisclosure testing, it can be determined whether the fetus is at 50% risk (because of having inherited a gene marker from the affected grandparent) or at very little risk (having inherited a gene marker from the unaffected grandparent). This is explained in more detail in appendix 5.

Nondisclosure prenatal testing requires the prospective parents to make difficult decisions if the test results indicate that the fetus is at 50% risk. Most prospective parents who request such testing intend to abort such a fetus. If the at-risk parent never gets HD, the couple will have aborted a normal fetus. On the other hand, if the at-risk parent does become affected and the fetus is not aborted, the parents will know that their child is highly likely to have HD. This choice puts the parents in the position of choosing that their child have testing without the child's consent. The knowledge that their child will get HD could cause difficult problems for both the affected and the unaffected parent and thereby for the child.

Testing At-Risk Persons Who Have an Affected Grandparent

Testing individuals who have an affected grandparent (i.e., who are at 25% risk or less) provides the same type of information as nondisclosure prenatal testing. The actual risk to the grandchild of an affected person will depend on the age of the person's parent (the offspring of the affected person). Even if the test outcome indicates that the grandchild is at risk, the risk may be less than 50% if the grandchild's parent is 45 years old or older. As explained in chapter 7, the risk for HD decreases steadily after age 45.

In the case of the grandchild of an affected person whose at-risk parent has died before living through the age of risk, nondisclosure testing may provide the only information it is possible to give.

Summary and Conclusions

Persons at risk for HD carry a variety of burdens. They may have the HD gene, and this may have direct cognitive or emotional consequences. Even if they do not have the gene, they may live most of their lives surrounded by family members with HD and the fear that they could become ill at any time. Given these unusual burdens, persons at risk for HD live surprisingly normal lives unless and until they develop symptoms of HD. A few at-risk persons request psychotherapy to help them deal with their burdens. Some burdens may also be lessened by certain aspects of genetic counseling.

Several years before it is possible for any physician to make a definite diagnosis, at-risk persons with the HD gene may have a depressed, irritable, or anxious mood or minor neurologic signs.

Genetic testing is now possible for some persons at risk, using genetic linkage analysis. Preliminary results from the few centers doing testing suggest that persons who have negative tests (are highly unlikely to have HD) are considerably relieved and those with positive tests (highly likely to have HD) cope fairly well, at least in the short term.

Appendix 1

The Documentation of Clinical Features of Huntington's Disease: Clinical Assessment Instruments

THE QUANTIFIED NEUROLOGICAL EXAMINATION (QNE)

Lateral Gaze

Pursuit: Hold index finger or pointer about 18″ from the patient's eye and ask him to follow it as it is *slowly* moved laterally.

Range:
  0 = normal
  1 = incomplete
  2 = no pursuit

Smoothness of movement:
  0 = one continuous movement
  1 = "catch" or jerky; may stop midmovement and look away from the target
  2 = no pursuit

Vertical Gaze

Pursuit: As the patient moves his eyes up and down, it is useful for the examiner to hold the eyelids up for a better view of smoothness and range of motion.

Range:
  0 = normal
  1 = incomplete
  2 = no pursuit

Smoothness of movement:
  0 = one continuous movement
  1 = "catch" or jerky movement
  2 = no pursuit

Saccades

Examiner holds up both index fingers about 18" from the patient at the extremes of lateral gaze and asks the patient to look from one finger to the other as quickly as possible, without moving the head.

Speed:

    0 = normal

    1 = slow

    2 = cannot execute command

Blink suppression:

(If the patient blinks while performing saccades, ask the patient to stop.)

    0 = does not blink or can stop

    1 = cannot stop blinking during saccades

    2 = cannot execute command

Smoothness of movement:

    0 = one smooth lateral movement

    1 = attains goal by series of short movements

    2 = cannot execute command

Head moves laterally:

(If the patient moves his head while performing saccades, ask the patient to stop.)

    0 = no head movement or can stop head movement

    1 = head moves with eyes

    2 = cannot do saccades

Gaze Holding

Ask the patient to focus on a target at the lateral extreme of gaze, about 18" away.

    0 = keeps eyes firmly on the target

    1 = eyes keep wandering off the target

    2 = cannot do saccades

Forceful Eye Closure

Ask the patient to close eyes tight; bury eyelids. Score normal if patient does so even momentarily.

    0 = buries lids

    1 = cannot bury lids

    2 = cannot execute command

Facial Mimicking

Ask the patient to mimic the examiner's performance of the following movements.

    0 = can perform

    1 = cannot perform

a. Blow out both cheeks at once, keeping mouth closed.

b. Put tongue in cheek with enough force to make the cheek "pouch out."

c. Frown (knit brows).
d. Wink (nonwinking eye may move but not close).
e. Rapid tongue movements. Ask the patient to touch the tip of his tongue to each corner of his lips alternately. Should be at least 4 touches/second and rhythmic to score 0.

Motor Impersistence

This item rates the patient's ability to sustain voluntary movement.
a. Eye closure. Ask the patient to close the eyes and keep them closed.
    0 = maintains eyes closed 20 seconds
    1 = opens eyes before 20 seconds
    2 = cannot execute command
b. Tongue. Ask the patient to protrude the tongue. It may not be held out by using the teeth.
    0 = maintains tongue out 20 seconds
    1 = opens before 20 seconds
    2 = cannot execute command

Speech: Repeated Syllables

Ask the patient to repeat the following syllables after the examiner.
Rhythm (rh):
    0 = regular
    1 = irregular
Rate (ra):
    0 = >4 syllables/sec
    1 = 4 syllables/sec or less
Clarity (cl):
    0 = each syllable clear
    1 = syllables run together
Add 1 to each category if mute (total = 12 if mute).
a. La-la-la . . .
b. Go-go-go . . .
c. Kitty-kitty-kitty . . .
d. Attenuation (ask the patient to count to 20—or score if noted in conversation).
    0 = no
    1 = yes
    2 = mute

Conversational Speech

This should be rated during the interview and examination.
Rhythm:
    0 = smooth with expected pauses and transitions
    1 = unexpected pauses; speech comes in bursts
    2 = mute

Rate:

   0 = normal speed

   1 = speech either too fast or too slow

   2 = mute

Clarity:

   0 = speech is normally understandable

   1 = examiner must listen carefully but does not need to ask the patient to repeat

   2 = patient must try more than once but can be understood

   3 = speech is almost or entirely incomprehensible

   4 = mute

Tone:

Examine tone in wrists and elbows.

   0 = normal

   1 = decreased

   2 = increased

Strength

Test biceps and strength of hand grasp unless more extensive examination is indicated.

   0 = normal

   1 = decreased

Deep Tendon Reflexes

Score the composite score of biceps, knees, and ankle jerks.

   0 = normal (1+, 2+)

   1 = absent

   2 = very brisk but no clonus

   3 = brisk with clonus at the ankle (or throughout)

(If asymmetrical, draw diagram on coding sheet showing findings.)

Plantar Response

For this reflex, score left and right responses separately.

   0 = flexor

   1 = extensor

Asymmetry

Tone, strength, DTRs.

   0 = all symmetrical

   1 = asymmetry present

(If code "1," describe on coding sheet.)

Finger-Nose

Ask the patient to point a finger and touch the examiner's finger and then the patient's own nose. The examiner's finger should be held far enough away so that the patient must completely extend the arm.

- 0 = quick, rhythmic, accurate (finger-nose-finger in one second)
- 1 = slow but accurate
- 2 = dysmetria
- 3 = cannot execute command

Finger-Thumb Tap

Ask the patient to tap the index or third finger with the thumb quickly. Score each hand separately.

- 0 = >4 taps/sec and rhythmic
- 1 = 3 taps/sec or faster but arrhythmic
- 2 = <3 taps/sec
- 3 = cannot perform

Diadochokinesis

Ask the patient to pronate and supinate the hand alternately, patting the other palm.
Score each hand separately.

- 0 = >3 pats/sec and rhythmic
- 1 = 2 pats/sec or faster but arrhythmic
- 2 = <2 pats/sec

Ask the patient to stand with feet together, eyes closed, arms out 90°, palms down, fingers apart. Note balance as well as any tremor or chorea of the fingertips. Score tremor or chorea.

Tremor

If the patient cannot stand, have the patient hold the arms at 90° while sitting. Tremor will not be scorable in patients with severe chorea.

- 0 = none
- 1 = mild
- 2 = marked
- 8 = cannot test because of chorea or poor concentration

Chorea

Notice all body parts and make a summary rating. Chorea is a fairly jerky movement that is not so stereotyped as a tic. It may be of any amplitude.

- 0 = absent
- 1 = mild, occasional
- 2 = frequent but low amplitude
- 3 = frequent or continuous with moderate amplitude
- 4 = continuous, severe, but the patient can carry out some voluntary movements

5 = so severe as to be totally incapacitating

Note: All patients should have chorea scored at rest and with stress.
Score as above in the following situations:

a. with arms extended forward at 90°, palms down, fingers spread.
b. in a relaxed position (sitting or lying down) and asked to try to stop all movement.
c. during conversation.
d. during voluntary movement (e.g., walking).
e. during stress (e.g., calculating).

Posture

(Rate standing or seated if the patient is unable to stand.)

0 = normal
1 = somewhat stooped
2 = very stooped, downward gaze or rigid and extended

Standing

Ask the patient to stand with feet touching, hands at the side.

0 = normally still or slight weaving
1 = widened base to stay in one place, or weaves excessively
2 = cannot stand still for 10 seconds or cannot stand

Now ask the patient to walk down a hallway. During the walking, ask the patient to stop, then continue, then turn around and come back. The requests to stop and turn around should be unexpected by the patient.

Walking

0 = normal gait, narrow base (heels should approximate a straight line)
1 = wide base
2 = wide base with deviation from a straight line
3 = walks with assistance (person, walker, leans on wall)
4 = unable to walk

Stopping

0 = stops on command
1 = stops but body lurches forward or takes a step
2 = takes 2 or more steps before stopping
3 = unable to walk

Turning

0 = pivots on a narrow base
1 = hesitates, widens base, and turns on two feet
2 = turns slowly and awkwardly
3 = cannot walk

Tandem Walk

Four practice steps, then 10 paces, heel touching toe at each step.

0 = no deviations or weaving after practice

1 = 1–3 deviations or excessive truncal weaving
2 = >3 deviations, but completes 10 paces
3 = cannot complete the task although tries
4 = cannot attempt task

Snout
Tap middle of closed lips with reflex hammer. Do not score random choreic movement.
    0 = absent
    1 = present

Grasp
Stroke the patient's palm, with the patient's palm down. Ask the patient not to grasp the examiner's hand.
    0 = absent
    1 = patient grasps examiner's hand

Bradykinesia
    0 = voluntary movements are performed at normal speed
    1 = mild slowness of gait, speech, task completion
    2 = marked slowness
    3 = in bed without voluntary movement

The Motor Impairment Scale (MIS) of the QNE
Eye closure (0–2); clarity of repeated syllables (0–4); finger-nose (0–3); diadochokinesis: right (0–3), left (0–3); plantar response (0–2); gait (0–4); tandem walk (0–4); bradykinesia (0–3). Maximum score = 28.

The Chorea Scale of the QNE
Chorea during: arm extentions (0–5); relaxation (0–5); conversation (0–5); voluntary movement (0–5); stress (0–5). Maximum score = 25.

The Eye Movement Scale of the QNE
Range of lateral gaze (0–2); smoothness of lateral movement (0–2); range of vertical gaze (0–2); smoothness of vertical movement (0–2); saccade speed (0–2); blink suppression during saccades (0–2); smoothness of saccadic movements (0–2); lateral head movement during saccades (0–2); gaze holding (0–2); forceful eye closure (0–2). Maximum score = 20.

THE MINI-MENTAL STATE EXAMINATION (MMSE)

Orientation
(1) Ask for the date. Then ask specifically for the parts omitted, e.g., "Can you also tell me what season it is?" One point for each correct answer.

(2) Ask in turn "Can you tell me the name of this hospital?" (town, county etc.). One point for each correct answer.

Registration

Ask the patient if you may do a memory test. Then say, clearly and slowly, the names of three unrelated objects, about one second for each. After you have said all three, ask the patient to repeat them. This first repetition determines the score (0–3), but keep saying them until the patient can repeat all three, up to six trials. If the patient does not eventually learn all three, recall cannot be meaningfully tested.

Attention and Calculation

Ask the patient to begin with 100 and count backward by 7. Stop after five subtractions (93, 86, 79, 72, 65). Score the total number of correct answers (e.g., "93, 88, 81, 74, 66" would give a score of 3). If the patient cannot or will not perform this task, ask the patient to spell the word *world* backward. The score is the number of letters in the correct order (e.g., dlrow = 5, dlorw = 3).

For purposes of following HD patients serially, it is best not to switch from serial sevens to spelling *world* backward when the patient will no longer perform serial sevens. This often elevates the MMSE score. The practice in the BHDP Research Clinic is to use serial sevens unless the patient has less than an eighth-grade education.

Recall

Ask the patient to recall the three words you previously asked to have remembered. Score 0–3.

Language

Naming: Show the patient a wristwatch and ask what it is. Repeat with a pencil. Score 0–2.

Repetition: Ask the patient to repeat the sentence after you. Allow only one trial. Score 0 or 1.

Three-stage Command: After gaining the patient's attention, repeat the command and then offer a blank sheet of paper. Be sure the paper is presented at the midline (i.e., neither toward the right hand nor toward the left hand). Score one point for each part correctly executed. Score 0–3.

Reading: On a blank sheet of paper, print the sentence "Close your eyes" in letters large enough for the patient to see clearly. Ask the patient to read it and do what it says. Score one point only if the patient actually closes the eyes. Score 0 or 1.

Writing: Give the patient a blank piece of paper and ask the patient to write a sentence for you. Do not dictate a sentence; it is to be written spontaneously. It must contain a subject and a verb and must be sensible. Correct punctuation and grammar are not necessary. Score 0 or 1.

Copying: On a blank sheet of paper, draw intersecting pentagons, each side about 1″ long, and ask the patient to copy it exactly. All 10 angles must be present and 2 must intersect to score 1 point. Tremor and rotation are ignored. Score 0 or 1.

Estimate the patient's level of sensorium along a continuum, from alert on the left to coma on the right.

		Maximum Score
Orientation		
What is the: (year) (season) (date) (day) (month)?	( )	5
Where are we: (state) (county or street) (town) (hospital) (floor)?	( )	5
Registration		
Name three objects: (one second to say each). Then ask the patient all three after you have said them. Give one point for each correct answer. Then repeat them until the patient learns all three. Count trials and record.	( )	3
Attention and Calculation		
Serial sevens. One point for each correct subtraction. Stop after five answers. Alternatively, spell *world* backward.	( )	5
Recall		
Ask for the three objects repeated above. Give one point for each correct answer.	( )	3
Language		
Name a pencil and a watch.	( )	2
Repeat the following: "No if's, and's, or but's."	( )	1
Follow a three-stage command: "Take a piece of paper in your right hand, fold it in half, and put it on the floor."	( )	3
Read and perform the following: "Close your eyes."	( )	1
Copy the interlocking pentagons.	( )	1
		Total Score

Assess the patient's level of consciousness along a continuum:
   Alert   Drowsy   Stupor   Coma

DOCUMENTATION OF ONSET OF SYMPTOMS: A SUGGESTED PROCEDURE

The documentation of the onset of signs and symptoms of HD is at best an estimate and can be approached in several ways. The most conservative approach (because it utilizes a sign instead of a symptom) is to date the onset from the time motor signs can be documented. However, as many as half the patients have reported changes in affect or behavior before the onset of motor abnormalities, so using motor signs in these cases results in a falsely late age at onset. The disadvantage of using behavioral and affective symptoms is that there are many other reasons for these symptoms in persons at risk in addition to the onset of HD. Therefore, when an at-risk person presents to a physician with changes in only affect or behavior, a diagnosis of HD cannot be confidently made.

Behavioral and affective symptoms can be used if the diagnosis is already clear, and onset information is being gathered in retrospect, for the purpose of estimating the duration of the illness for a disability application or prognosticating about length of life. Documenting the earliest noticeable sign or symptom of whatever type is also important in genetic counseling. Because of the positive correlation of the age at onset in family members, the remaining risk for an asymptomatic family member can be more accurately estimated if the age at onset of several affected family members is documented.

In the BHDP Clinic, we developed a sequence of questions that seems to be useful in documenting onset retrospectively. This method is reliable between interviewers but has not been tested using more than one family informant, because two equally knowledgeable informants are rarely available.

1. Document the family history, which will include names and birth and death dates for the patient's sibs, spouse, and children.
2. Ask the best available informant (who should have been living with or near the patient at the time of onset): "As you look back on it, when do you think ——'s symptoms first started?"
3. The informant will guess a certain year. Then, using the pedigree, remind the informant of some family event that took place at that time (e.g., the birth of a child or grandchild). Ask where they were living, or what job the patient or spouse had at that time. These questions will allow the informant to put the guessed year in context, which often results in a revision of the estimate.
4. If the informant mentioned a motor sign, ask if any cognitive, behavioral, or affective changes preceded that, and vice versa.
5. The following examples may help the informant understand the kinds of things that may represent early motor, cognitive, and affective manifestations of HD.

Examples of Early Manifestations of Motor Abnormalities
Uneven pressure on the gas pedal of the car
Ticlike movements of fingers, face, feet, or shoulders
Restless or fidgetiness of whole body or feet while seated
Unexplained falls
Clumsiness with tools or household appliances

Examples of Early Manifestations of Cognitive Problems
Decline in efficiency of planning and executing a work plan (at home, in school, or in employment)
Slowness or inaccuracy in balancing checkbook
Forgetfulness about appointments or chores
Vagueness in conversation

Examples of Affective or Behavioral Change
Increasing irritability with the family or a longer duration of anger when it occurs
Decline in interest in household tasks or social events
Increasing anxiety over seemingly trivial issues or decisions
An episode of major depression or mania

THE ACTIVITIES OF DAILY LIVING: A QUESTIONNAIRE DEVELOPED FOR HD

Name of patient: _____

Name of informant: _____

Date: _____

Instructions: The following information should be supplied by the spouse, caretaker, or whoever knows the patient or person at risk best. If, at the present time, there is no opportunity for a particular task because the patient is in the hospital, circle the answer that best fits your appraisal of the patient's ability. Persons at risk, even though perfectly able to answer the questions, should have a spouse/parent complete the form.

Item	0	1	2	3	8
Personal Care					
Eating	Normal	Independent but slow or some spills	Needs help to cut or pour; spills often, avoids some foods	Must be fed most foods	
Dressing	Normal	Slow or clumsy but independent	Needs help with ties, buttons, zippers	Needs help with all clothing	
Interest in personal appearance	Same as always	Interested if going out but not at home	Allows self to be groomed, or does on request	Resists efforts of caretaker to clean and groom	
Taking pills, medicines	Remembers without help	Remembers if dose left in special place	Tries but forgets often if not reminded	Medicine must be given by others	No regular pills
Household Care					
Cooking	Plans and prepares meals	Some cooking but less than normal	Gets food out if it is prepared by others	Does nothing to fix meals	
Housekeeping	Keeps house as usual	Does at least half of usual jobs	Occasional dusting or small jobs	No longer keeps house	Never did jobs
Home maintenance	Does all tasks as usual	Does at least half of usual tasks	Occasional raking or other minor jobs	No longer does any maintenance	Never did any
Home repairs	Does all usual repairs	Does at least half of usual repairs	Occasional, minor repairs	No longer does any repairs	Never did any
Work and Money					
Employment (outside home)	Doing as well as ever	Some trouble with job but still at same job	Works at easier job or part-time; trouble finding a job	No longer works at all	Never worked

Handling money	As well as usual	Trouble with checkbook or in making decisions about spending	Most management taken over by others	No longer handles money	
Social Relationships					
With spouse	As good as ever	Mild marital problems	Serious marital problems but still living together	Divorce or separation with no further relationship	Never married
With children	Adequate parent	More easily irritated; quicker to punish	Neglects their physical or emotional needs	Cannot care for children; abuses them	No children or grown before onset
Friends or other family members	Sees as often as ever	Sees less often	Accepts visitors or invitations but doesn't seek company	Refuses to socialize	
Keeping busy	Same interests as usual	Less interested but still does on occasion	Watches TV or watches others do things	If left alone, does nothing	
Communication					
Travel	Same as usual	Gets out if someone else drives	Gets out in wheelchair	Home or hospital bound	
Phone	Same as usual	Calls a few familiar numbers	Will answer phone only	Never uses a phone	Never had a phone
Write	Writes or types letters	Writes less often, or writes grocery list	May sign name, leave message	Never writes	Never wrote much

Appendix 2

DSM III-R Criteria for Psychiatric Disorders Commonly Seen in Huntington's Disease

(Extracted and revised from the American Psychiatric Association's *Diagnostic and Statistical Manual of Mental Disorders,* Third Edition Revised, reprinted with permission)

DIAGNOSTIC CRITERIA FOR SCHIZOPHRENIA

A. The presence of characteristic psychotic symptoms in the active phase: either (1), (2), or (3) for at least one week (unless the symptoms are successfully treated):
  (1) two of the following:
    (a) delusions
    (b) prominent hallucinations (throughout the day for several days or several times a week for several weeks, each hallucinatory experience not being limited to a few brief moments)
    (c) incoherence or marked loosening of associations
    (d) catatonic behavior
    (e) flat or grossly inappropriate affect
  (2) bizarre delusions (i.e., involving a phenomenon that the person's culture would regard as totally implausible, e.g., thought broadcasting, being controlled by a dead person)
  (3) prominent hallucinations [as defined in (1)(b) above] of a voice with content having no apparent relation to depression or elation, or a voice keeping up a running commentary on the person's behavior or thoughts, or two or more voices conversing with each other
B. Schizoaffective disorder and mood disorder with psychotic features have been ruled out, i.e., if a major depressive or manic syndrome has ever been present during an active phase of the disturbance, the total duration

of all episodes of a mood syndrome has been brief relative to the total duration of the active and residual phases of the disturbance.

C. Continuous signs of the disturbance for at least six months. The six-month period must include an active phase (of at least one week, or less if symptoms have been successfully treated) during which there were psychotic symptoms characteristic of schizophrenia (symptoms in A), with or without a prodromal or residual phase, as defined below. Prodromal/residual symptoms alone without an active phase are not sufficient for a diagnosis of schizophrenia.

PRODROMAL OR RESIDUAL SYMPTOMS (AT LEAST 2)

(1) marked social isolation or withdrawal
(2) marked impairment in role functioning as wage-earner, student, or home-maker
(3) markedly peculiar behavior (e.g., collecting garbage, talking to self in public, hoarding food)
(4) marked impairment in personal hygiene and grooming
(5) blunted or inappropriate affect
(6) digressive, vague, overelaborate, or circumstantial speech, or poverty of speech, or poverty of content of speech
(7) odd beliefs or magical thinking, influencing behavior and inconsistent with cultural norms, e.g., superstitious, belief in clairvoyance, telepathy, "sixth sense," "others can feel my feelings," overvalued ideas, ideas of reference
(8) unusual perceptual experiences, e.g., recurrent illusions, sensing the presence of a force or person not actually present
(9) marked lack of initiative, interests, or energy

DIAGNOSTIC CRITERIA FOR MANIC AND HYPOMANIC EPISODES

Note: A "manic syndrome" is defined as including criteria A, B, and C below. A "hypomanic syndrome" is defined as including criteria A and B, but not C, i.e., no marked impairment.

A. A distinct period of abnormally and persistently elevated, expansive, or irritable mood
B. During the period of mood disturbance, at least three of the following symptoms have persisted (four if the mood is only irritable) and have been present to a significant degree:
(1) inflated self-esteem or grandiosity
(2) decreased need for sleep, e.g., feels rested after only three hours of sleep

(3) more talkative than usual or pressure to keep talking

(4) flight of ideas or subjective experience that thoughts are racing

(5) distractibility, i.e., attention too easily drawn to unimportant or irrelevant external stimuli

(6) increase in goal-directed activity (either socially, at work or school, or sexually) or psychomotor agitation

(7) excessive involvement in pleasurable activities that have a high potential for painful consequences, e.g., the person engages in unrestrained buying sprees, sexual indiscretions, or foolish business investments

C. Mood disturbance sufficiently severe to cause marked impairment in occupational functioning or in usual social activities or relationships with others, or to necessitate hospitalization to prevent harm to self or others

D. At no time during the disturbance have there been delusions or hallucinations for as long as two weeks in the absence of prominent mood symptoms (i.e., before the mood symptoms developed or after they have remitted)

E. Not superimposed on schizophrenia, schizophreniform disorder, delusional disorder, or psychotic disorder NOS.

DIAGNOSTIC CRITERIA FOR MAJOR DEPRESSIVE EPISODE

Note: A "major depressive syndrome" is defined as criterion A below.

A. At least five of the following symptoms have been present during the same one-month period and represent a change from previous functioning; at least one of the symptoms is either (1) depressed mood, or (2) loss of interest or pleasure. (Do not include mood-incongruent delusions or hallucinations, incoherence, or marked loosening of associations.)

(1) depressed mood (or can be irritable mood in children and adolescents) most of the day, nearly every day, as indicated either by subjective account or observation by others

(2) markedly diminished interest or pleasure in all, or almost all, activities most of the day, nearly every day (as indicated either by subjective account or observation by others of apathy most of the time)

(3) significant weight loss or weight gain when not dieting (e.g., more than 5 percent of body weight in a month), or decrease or increase in appetite nearly every day (in children, consider failure to make expected weight gains)

(4) insomnia or hypersomnia nearly every day

(5) psychomotor agitation or retardation nearly every day (observable

by others, not merely subjective feelings of restlessness or being slowed down)

(6) fatigue or loss of energy nearly every day

(7) feelings of worthlessness or excessive inappropriate guilt (which may be delusional) nearly every day (not merely self-reproach or guilt about being sick)

(8) diminished ability to think or concentrate, or indecisiveness, nearly every day (either by subjective account or as observed by others)

(9) recurrent thoughts of death (not just fear of dying), recurrent suicidal ideation without a specific plan, or a suicide attempt or a specific plan for committing suicide

(10) depression regularly worse in the morning and there may also be early morning awakening (at least two hours before usual time of awakening)

B. The disturbance is not a normal reaction to the death of a loved one, (uncomplicated bereavement) diagnosis of Huntington's disease or loss of employment.

Note: Morbid preoccupation with worthlessness, suicidal ideation, marked functional impairment or psychomotor retardation, or prolonged duration suggest bereavement complicated by major depression.

C. At no time during the disturbance have there been delusions or hallucinations for as long as two weeks in the absence of prominent mood symptoms (i.e., before the mood symptoms developed or after they have remitted).

D. Not superimposed on schizophrenia, schizophreniform disorder, delusional disorder, or psychotic disorder NOS.

DIAGNOSTIC CRITERIA FOR 300.40 DYSTHYMIA

A. Depressed mood (or can be irritable mood in children and adolescents) for most of the day, more days than not, as indicated either by subjective account or observation by others, for at least two years (one year for children and adolescents)

B. Presence, while depressed, of at least two of the following:

(1) poor appetite or overeating

(2) insomnia or hypersomnia

(3) low energy or fatigue

(4) low self-esteem

(5) poor concentration or difficulty making decisions

(6) feelings of hopelessness

C. During a two-year period (one year for children and adolescents) of the disturbance, never without the symptoms in A for more than two months at a time

D. No evidence of an unequivocal major depressive episode during the first two years (one year for children and adolescents) of the disturbance. Note: There may have been a previous major depressive episode, provided there was a full remission (no significant signs or symptoms for six months) before the development of dysthymia. In addition, after these two years (one year in children and adolescents) of dysthymia, there may be superimposed episodes of major depression, in which case both diagnoses are given.
E. Has never had a manic episode or an unequivocal hypomanic episode
F. Not superimposed on a chronic psychotic disorder, such as schizophrenia or delusional disorder
G. It cannot be established that a medication initiated and maintained the disturbance, e.g., prolonged administration of an antihypertensive medication.

DIAGNOSTIC CRITERIA FOR 300.02 GENERALIZED ANXIETY DISORDER

A. Unrealistic or excessive anxiety and worry (apprehensive expectation) about two or more life circumstances, e.g., worry about possible misfortune to one's child (who is in no danger) and worry about finances (for no good reason), for a period of six months or longer, during which the person has been bothered more days than not by these concerns. In children and adolescents, this may take the form of anxiety and worry about academic, athletic, and social performance.
B. If another Axis I disorder is present, the focus of the anxiety and worry in A is unrelated to it, e.g., the anxiety or worry is not about having a panic attack (as in panic disorder), being embarrassed in public (as in social phobia), or gaining weight (as in anorexia nervosa).
C. This disturbance does not occur only during the course of a mood disorder or a psychotic disorder.
D. At least six of the following 18 symptoms are often present when anxious (do not include symptoms present only during panic attacks):
   Motor tension:
   (1) trembling, twitching, or feeling shaky
   (2) muscle tension, aches, or soreness
   (3) restlessness
   (4) easy fatigability
   Autonomic hyperactivity:
   (5) shortness of breath or smothering sensations
   (6) palpitations or accelerated heart rate (tachycardia)
   (7) sweating, or cold clammy hands
   (8) dry mouth
   (9) dizziness or lightheadedness

(10) nausea, diarrhea, or other abdominal distress
(11) flushes (hot flashes) or chills
(12) frequent urination
(13) trouble swallowing or "lump in throat"
Vigilance and scanning:
(14) feeling keyed up or on edge
(15) exaggerated startle response
(16) difficulty concentrating or "mind going blank" because of anxiety
(17) trouble falling or staying asleep
(18) irritability
E. It cannot be established that an organic factor (other than Huntington's disease) initiated and maintained the disturbance, e.g., hyperthyroidism, caffeine intoxication.

DIAGNOSTIC CRITERIA FOR 312.34 INTERMITTENT EXPLOSIVE DISORDER

A. Several discrete episodes of loss of control of aggressive impulses resulting in assaultive acts or destruction of property.
B. The degree of aggressiveness expressed during the episodes is grossly out of proportion to any precipitating psychosocial stressors.
C. There are no signs of generalized impulsiveness or aggressiveness between the episodes. In fact, patients may be generally apathetic.
D. The episodes of loss of control do not occur during the course of a psychotic disorder, antisocial or borderline personality disorder, conduct disorder, or intoxication with a psychoactive substance.

Appendix 3

Developing Large Kindreds: Genealogic Strategies

REASONS FOR WISHING TO FIND LARGE KINDREDS

One purpose of genetic counseling for persons at risk for HD is to estimate the remaining risk for developing HD. This estimate is made more accurate by knowing the sex of the affected parent and the mean and distribution of the age at onset of many relatives. Developing a large kindred is too time consuming for most clinics, but the person at risk can be taught how to accomplish most of the research himself. A second reason to develop large kindreds is to ascertain persons at risk. This would be important if there were an effective medical treatment or prevention for HD. Many persons are unaware of their risk for HD and could not take advantage of treatment unless they were found through genealogic investigation of affected and unaffected relatives. Finally, large kindreds have been required to carry out genetic linkage analysis and other kinds of genetic research.

For this last purpose, it is necessary first to find promising families, most of whose members live within reasonable distance of the investigation site. If clinical examination and blood-drawing are required for many family members, long distances lead to unreasonable expenses and are often associated with looser family ties and thus more difficulty in gaining cooperation. Promising families can be identified in two ways. Occasionally, such a family appears in a clinic or is reported by a social or caregiving agency. A sure way to find large families is in a state-wide survey of HD. Several branches of large families will be found independently, each branch unaware of the others but with surnames or relatives in common. By developing a surname index, the investigator can usually link these branches together into much larger kindreds.

Once the outline of a kindred is sketched out, the same genealogic tactics are used as described for more limited genealogic investigations, except that more informants and more medical records are required. In addition, other genealogic sources, such as census data, wills, and birth and death certificates, are helpful (Hawkins, Murphy, and Abbey 1965).

To construct large pedigrees, it is useful to find a family genealogist and family leaders. It has been surprising in our genealogic work how often a family member is found who has already researched the family tree and can provide correct names, birth names, and birth and death dates. This person will not necessarily know which members of the kindred had HD, but the available information will provide access to records (e.g., death certificates) that contain diagnostic information and place of death, which in turn lead to medical records. Some family genealogists have copies of death certificates and obituaries that can give clues as to who was affected, as well as the names of offspring. Family genealogists will often be willing to undertake further research and can become valuable collaborators.

In addition to a family genealogist, it is helpful to identify family leaders for each branch of the family. These individuals are usually unaffected persons at risk for HD or spouses of affected members. They are motivated to help at-risk relatives contact distantly related family members. They see the value of genetic counseling and research projects, usually have a good understanding of the goal, and have the confidence of their close family members. These family leaders will know how best to approach relatives and can help avoid damaging family relationships.

When attempting to construct a large kindred, it is sometimes useful for an investigator to screen medical records in certain hospitals for surnames in addition to requesting individual medical records on persons suspected by informants to have HD. Until very recently, many HD patients were admitted to public psychiatric hospitals. Now they more often go to nursing homes, which have extremely poor records, no surname or diagnostic indexing system, and very poor quality diagnostic information. However, for patients in earlier generations (from the late 1800s through the 1970s), public psychiatric hospital records provide valuable diagnostic and genealogic information. Review of medical records for research purposes requires a research protocol approved both by one's own institution and by the hospital in question. For clinical purposes it is necessary only to have a family member sign a request for release of information and the devoted cooperation of the record librarian. Explain the reasons for the request to the librarian and attempt to arouse interest; a willingness to search for records can decide the success of the search.

In the nomenclature and indexing system used by psychiatric hospitals, HD is not recorded as a separate diagnosis, so a search for all HD records is not possible. In the psychiatric statistical manuals, HD is subsumed under "organic brain syndrome" or "primary degenerative dementia," and only a tiny minority of the patients so categorized will have HD. For an individual kindred, however, it is possible to obtain permission to search the surname index at the hospitals serving the towns where most of the family lived. This should be done after a fairly substantial pedigree has been constructed, so that many surnames are known. The surname index should be searched for both affected and reportedly unaffected lines.

When reviewing the case notes located by the search, the investigator will find a variety of irrelevant diagnoses. Disregard these, and scan each chart for descriptions of involuntary movement and a gradual deterioration in gait, cognition, and the ability to swallow food. These are usually best documented in the nursing notes. The social work notes ordinarily provide the best family history; names and health status of parents and siblings will normally be described therein, and sometimes addresses and birth dates are recorded.

OTHER GENEALOGIC RESOURCES FOR ESTABLISHING LARGE KINDREDS

While public records do not provide accurate medical information, they can provide names, birth names, and birth and death dates that will facilitate the search for medical records. Start with the current generation and work back in time. The death certificates of any members of recent generations will provide a birth date and names of the person's parents. The exact death date (usually provided by a family Bible or other personal records) must be provided to obtain the death certificate. These names and dates will provide enough information to search the appropriate *National Decennial Census* for the nuclear family. Census listings between 1790 and 1840 list heads of household by name and enumerate all other family members by number only. From 1850, the census lists the head of household and all residents by name, age, race, sex, education, and occupation. Real property is listed, which allows a search of the head of household's will. We have occasionally used wills, obituaries, church registries, and the records maintained by funeral directors. Other documents are available at state historical societies, and the society's staff, as well as local librarians, can suggest other sources for a particular surname.

In summary, it is possible with a systematic effort to construct the very large HD kindreds necessary for some clinical and research purposes. However, less extensive though similar genealogic investigation is often adequate to establish or rule out the diagnosis of HD. Where clinical resources are insufficient to carry out such investigations, family members, with instruction, can often provide considerable assistance to the medical staff.

Appendix 4

Service Organizations and Agencies

VOLUNTARY ORGANIZATIONS

Australia:	Australian Huntington's Disease Association P.O. Box 7, Killara 2071, New South Wales, Australia
Belgium:	Huntington Liga Krykelberg 1, 3043 Bierbeek, Belgium 6 De Dries, B2130 Brasschaat, Belgium
Great Britain:	Association to Combat Huntington's Chorea Borough House, 34A Station Road, Hinckley, Leics LE10 1AP England
Canada:	Huntington Society of Canada Box 333, Cambridge, Ontario N1R 5T8, Canada
Denmark:	Landsforeningen mod Huntington's Chorea Blegdamsvej 3, DK-2200 Copenhagen N., Denmark
France:	Association Huntington de France Residence Manin, 119 rue Manin, 75019 Paris, France
Ireland:	Huntington's Disease Association of Ireland 279 Sutton Park, Dublin 13, Ireland
Italy:	Associazione por Combattere la Corea di Huntington Instituto Neurologico 'C Besta' Via Coloria 11, Milano 20133, Italy 24 Parco Margherita, Napoli 80121, Italy
The Netherlands:	Vereniging van Huntington Postbus 30470, 2500 GL s'Gravenhage, Netherlands
New Zealand:	New Zealand Huntington's Disease Association 23 Konene Street, Roturua, New Zealand

Norway:	Landsforeningen for Huntingtons Sykdom Department of Social Medicine, Rikshospitalet, Oslo 1, Norway
South Africa:	Professor Beighton Department of Human Genetics, University of Capetown Medical School, Observatory 7925, Cape Town, South Africa
United States:	Huntington's Disease Society of America, Inc. 140 W. 22nd Street, 6th floor, New York, NY 10011, USA Toll free number: 1-800-345-HDSA
West Germany:	Huntington Gruppen in der Familienholfe eV. Bahnhofstr. 7A, 3550 Marburg, West Germany

BRAIN BANKS

Brain Tissue Resource Center
McLean Hospital
115 Mill Street
Belmont, MA 02178–9983
Telephone: (617) 855–2400

Dr. Tourtellote, Chief, Neurology Service
Director, National Neurological Research Bank
Veterans Administration Wadsworth Medical Center
Wilshire and Sawtelle Blvds.
Los Angeles, CA 90073

NATIONAL HD ROSTER AND DNA BANK

Huntington's Disease Research Roster
Department of Medical Genetics
Indiana University School of Medicine
1100 W. Michigan Street
Indianapolis, IN 46223
Telephone: (317) 264-2241

Appendix 5

Genetic Issues

ESTIMATION OF GENETIC RISK

Age-at-Onset Distribution for Maternally and Paternally Transmitted HD for Use in Genetic Counseling

Because of the paternal transmission effect, the age-at-onset distribution differs somewhat for the offspring of affected mothers and affected fathers (figure app5.1A). From the point of view of genetic counseling, the risk for HD to an asymptomatic offspring of a parent with HD decreases slightly earlier for the offspring of affected fathers (figure app5.1B). See also chapter 7.

GENETIC NOTATION

Using genetic notation facilitates the efficient and accurate documentation of family structure. Figure App5.2 illustrates the most frequently used symbols. See also chapter 8. More detailed instructions for genetic notation can be found in Jorgenson, Yoder, and Shapiro 1980.

GENETIC TESTING FOR HD

In different families, different marker types are on the same chromosome with HD. Each family has to be tested individually to determine which marker is near the HD gene for that family. For this reason, blood must be collected from the person requesting testing and several family members, some affected and some unaffected with HD. DNA is then extracted from the blood leukocytes of each family member. DNA can also be extracted from frozen brain, fibroblasts, or any other frozen tissue that may be available from deceased family members.

As illustrated in figure app5.3, the DNA from each family member is cut into fragments (or digested) by a restriction enzyme or endonuclease, and the

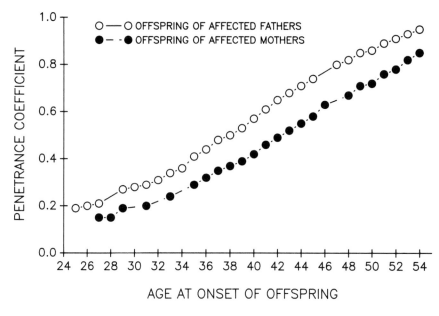

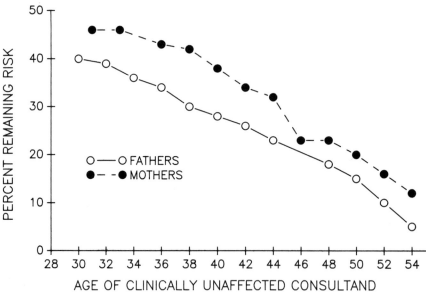

Figure App5.1. Age-at-onset distribution for maternally (filled circles) and paternally (open circles) transmitted HD. Adapted from Chase et al. 1986.

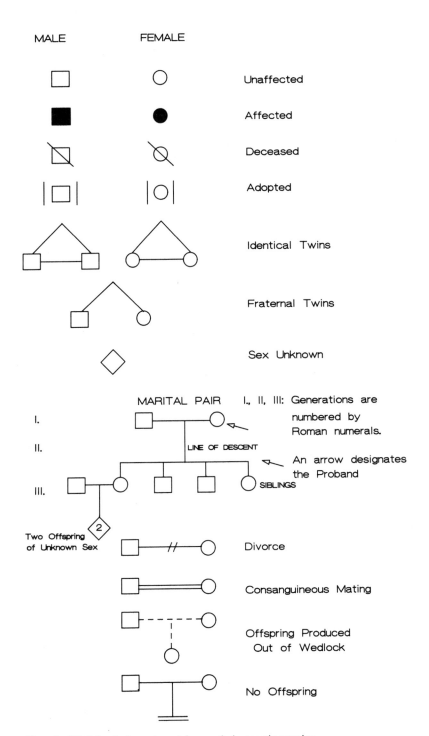

Figure App5.2. 0 Symbols used most frequently in genetic notation.

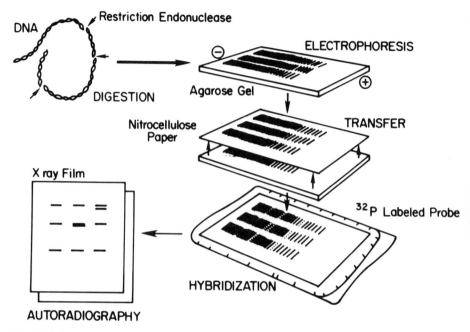

Figure App5.3. The Southern Blotting Process. See text for explanation. This figure was kindly provided by Dr. Haig H. Kazazian.

fragments are spread apart along a gel column by an electrical current passing through the gel containing the DNA fragments (electrophoresis). The longer DNA fragments will move along the gel more slowly than the short ones, so they will be spread out according to size, with progressively smaller fragments moving toward the bottom of the column.

The restriction enzyme cuts the DNA wherever a certain sequence of nucleotides occurs. For example, the Hind-III enzyme cuts DNA at every AAGCTT sequence along the human genome. If a mutation occurs anywhere along such a sequence of nucleotides (changing the sequence, for example, to AAGGTT), the enzyme will no longer recognize it as a cut site, and the DNA will not be cut there.

The enzyme chosen to cut the DNA of the family members into fragments depends on which marker is being used. The G8 marker (D4S10), the first marker discovered to be linked to the HD gene, is made from a piece of human DNA near the HD gene where there are two recognition sites for the enzyme Hind-III (and several others). However, these sites are present in some persons but not in others. That is, two Hind-III recognition sites are *polymorphic* along the length of DNA from which the G8 marker was made.

After the DNA fragments from the family members have been separated on the columns, the column of fragments is transferred to paper (figure app5.3). The marker (or probe) is made radioactive and the paper with the family's DNA fragments on it is soaked in a solution containing the radioactive marker. The marker will stick to (hybridize with) the DNA fragments from chromosome 4 that are its complement. It will not stick to any other DNA. The number of DNA fragments the marker sticks to depends on how many Hind-III recognition sites are present from the area of chromosome 4 that the marker recognizes. The hybridized radioactive marker fragments are visualized by exposing the nitrocellulose paper to Xray film (autoradiography). Wherever the marker sticks, a thin radioactive line will appear on the column of DNA fragments. In other words, the pattern of radioactive lines (or bands) will vary from person to person depending on the number of Hind-III recognition sites (and consequently the number of DNA fragments) that the marker sticks to. This is called the Southern blotting process, named for the person who developed it.

Next, the geneticist and the genetic analyst doing the test will "read" the patterns for all the affected and unaffected family members and try to deduce the marker pattern of the affected members. The marker types assigned to each family member are entered into a computer program, such as LIPED (Ott 1974), which calculates the probability that the person requesting the testing has the HD gene.

In the first example given below (figure app5.4A), the affected family members have a $+/-$ pattern at the PstI site of the G8 probe, while the escapee aunt (2.5) of the person requesting testing has the $-/-$ pattern. Combining this information with the patterns of the grandmother (1.2) and the unaffected mother (2.6), the genetic counselor could predict that the young man requesting the testing (3.3) has inherited the HD gene, while his sister has not. The second example (figure app5.4B) illustrates the two polymorphic Hind-III sites of the same G8 probe, and the increased number of possible marker patterns when there are two polymorphic sites (bottom of figure). This example is complicated by the fact that all three affected family members (1.3, 1.5, and 2.1) share both patterns. However, 2.1 could have only inherited the $+/+$ pattern from her deceased affected father, because her mother is homozygous for the $-/+$ pattern. The young woman requesting the testing did not inherit the $+/+$ pattern from her mother, so she is highly unlikely to have inherited the HD gene.

Here are several examples of families who have been informative for testing, and one family who was not informative. Instead of $+/-$, each Southern blot pattern has been assigned a letter for clarity. Some diagrams represent real families whose structure has been altered to preserve confidentiality; others have been created to serve as illustrations.

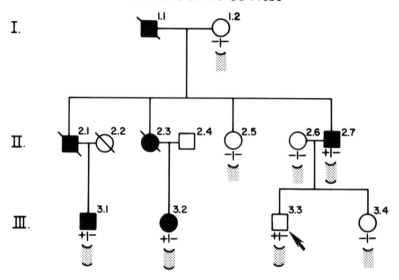

An HD Family that is Informative for the Polymorphic Pst I Site of the G8 Probe

Possible Marker Patterns for the One Polymorphic Pst I Site

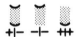

Figure App5.4. *Above and opposite;* in these two families a person at risk (designated by an arrow) requested presymptomatic testing. Because the markers distinguished a particular pattern associated with the HD gene it was possible to provide an accurate estimate of risk to the persons at risk who requested the information. See also text and chapter 10.

Example 1

In this example (figure app5.5) the father and paternal aunt of the at-risk son both have HD. The father inherited the B marker from the unaffected grand-mother; therefore, he inherited the C marker from his deceased affected grand-father. Using similar reasoning, we can say that the aunt also inherited the C marker from her deceased grandfather.

If the at-risk son inherits the C marker from his affected father (making him either CA or CD), he will likely develop HD. If he inherits the B marker from his father (making his marker type BA or BD), he will probably not develop HD, because the B marker came from his unaffected grandmother.

An HD Family that is Informative for the Polymorphic Hind Ⅲ Sites of the G8 Probe

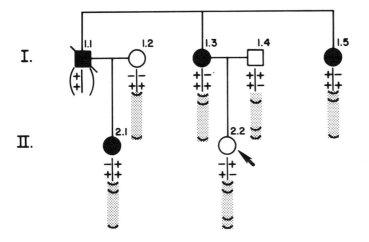

Possible Marker Patterns for the Two Hind Ⅲ Sites

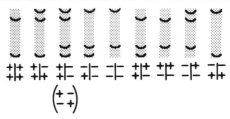

Fig. 5-4B

Example 2

If an unaffected grandparent is available, an at-risk person can sometimes be tested if only one affected close relative is available.

In this example (figure app5.6), the only affected person available for chromosomal analysis is the affected mother. However, her son and daughter can be tested, because their unaffected grandmother is living. Because the mother, AB, and the escapee aunt, AA, could inherit only an A marker from the grandmother, the affected mother must have inherited the B marker from the deceased affected grandfather. Therefore, we infer that the B marker is linked to HD in this family. By knowing the father's markers, we can deduce that the at-risk daughter (CA) is unlikely to have inherited HD, while the at-risk son (AB) probably has inherited it and will become affected.

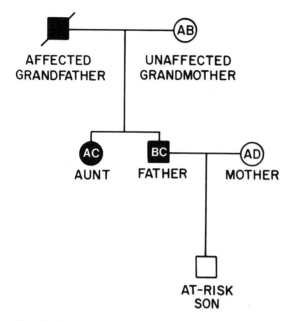

Figure App5.5. Example pedigree #1.

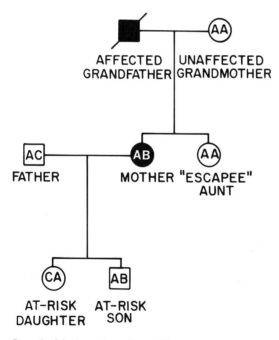

Figure App5.6. Example pedigree #2.

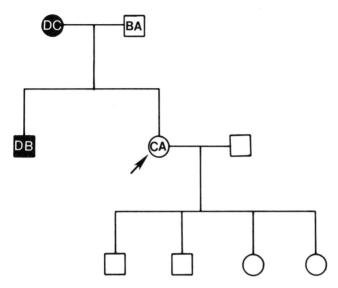

Figure App5.7. Example pedigree #3.

Example 3

This family (figure app5.7) illustrates the absolute minimum structure for doing genetic testing. Most families with this structure would be uninformative, but the at-risk woman in this family (the case example for chapter 10) could be told with 99% probability that she did not have the HD gene. This could be done because she and her brother inherited four different marker types. Their father's markers were known, and this allowed the investigator to infer the marker types of the deceased mother.

The examples above demonstrate that the marker type near the HD gene differs from one family to the next. In example 1 it was C, in example 2 it was B. This is why it is necessary to have blood from several *closely related* family members to do the test. For each family, the marker type near the HD gene must be established *in that family*.

Example 4: Uninformative Families

Some families will be uninformative for the marker test because DNA is not available from enough people in the family. At-risk persons from such families cannot be tested. For other families, or parts of families, the test will be uninformative because affected and unaffected relatives share the same marker types.

In example 4 (figure app5.8), although several relatives are available, the test test will not be informative because variety is lacking among the markers. In this family, A is the marker near the HD gene. The affected mother and affected aunt both have the AC pattern. We know from the escapee uncle and unaffected

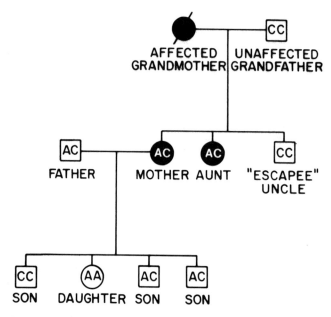

Figure App5.8. Example pedigree #4.

grandfather that the C marker is not linked to HD in this family. The AC mother has four at-risk children. However, the children's father also has markers A and C. For this reason, it will not be possible to determine whether the A that was inherited by an at-risk AC child came from the affected or the unaffected parent.

We can predict that the CC son will remain well. He inherited the father's C marker and the mother's C marker, which in this family is not near the HD gene. The AA daughter is likely to develop HD, because she inherited A from her mother as well as from her father. However, for the two sons with AC markers the test is uninformative; we cannot tell whether they inherited their father's A marker or their mother's A marker.

Example 5: Errors Related to Falsely Specified Paternity

Incorrect information about the identity of the at-risk person's biological father can sometimes be detected because the at-risk person has inherited a marker that neither parent has. However, in some cases, the falsely specified paternity is not detected and can lead to errors in testing.

In example 5 (figure app5.9), A is the marker near the HD gene. The at-risk son being tested assumes that the man with marker pattern CC is his father. His test results indicate that he inherited the A marker from his affected mother, predicting that he too will be affected with HD. Actually, the man with marker type AA is his biological father. The at-risk son had to inherit the A marker

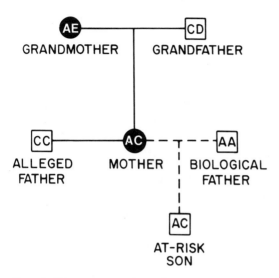

Figure App5.9. Example pedigree #5.

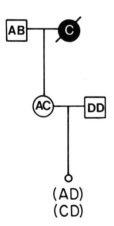

Figure App5.10. Example pedigree #6.

from his biological father and, therefore, the C marker from his mother. In reality, he will probably be unaffected.

Example 6: Prenatal Testing

The marker may be used for prenatal testing under two conditions: (1) when the potential parent has HD or has had a positive test for HD, *disclosure testing* may be carried out, and (2) when the potential parent is at risk for HD, *nondisclosure testing* is possible. Testing the fetus in the first instance is identical with pre-symptomatic testing, as explained above. The test will be either positive (the fetus is up to 99% likely to be affected), negative (the fetus is up to 99% likely to be unaffected), or uninformative.

However, in nondisclosure testing, the test outcomes are that the fetus may be either at very low risk (1% or less) or at the same risk as his at-risk parent, up to 50%, depending on the parent's age. The same applies to testing of persons at 25% risk, i.e., who have an affected grandparent.

In example 6 (figure app5.10), an at-risk mother and her husband wish to have a child, but they do not want to chance transmitting the HD gene. The mother cannot have presymptomatic testing because her affected parent is deceased and there are not enough other close relatives for testing to be informative. Because her unaffected father is living (markers A and B), and because the at-risk mother has a marker that he does not have, C, it can be deduced that the marker comes from her deceased affected mother. It cannot be determined whether that marker is the one near the HD gene or the one near the normal gene, but it is marker C that puts the mother at risk. Therefore, if the fetus inherits marker A from its mother, it is at very low risk (less than 1%) for having HD. If the fetus inherited marker C from its mother, it is at approximately 50% risk, like the mother.

References

Adams, R. D., and M. Victor, eds. 1985. *Principles of Neurology.* 3rd ed. New York: McGraw-Hill.

Albert, M. S., N. Butters, and J. Brandt. 1981a. Development of remote memory loss in patients with Huntington's disease. *Journal of Clinical Neuropsychology* 3:1–12.

Albert, M. S., N. Butters, and J. Brandt. 1981b. Patterns of remote memory in amnesic and demented patients. *Archives of Neurology* 38:495–500.

Albert, M. L., R. G. Feldman, and A. L. Willis. 1974. The 'subcortical dementia' of progressive supranuclear palsy. *Journal of Neurology, Neurosurgery, and Psychiatry* 37:121–30.

Alexander, G. E. 1984. Instruction-dependent neuronal activity in primate putamen. *Society for Neuroscience Abstracts* 10:515.

Alexander, G. E., M. R. DeLong, and P. L. Strick. 1986. Parallel organization of functionally segregated circuits linking basal ganglia and cortex. *Annual Review of Neuroscience* 9:357–81.

Alexander, G. E., E. D. Witt, and P. S. Goldman-Rakic. 1980. Neuronal activity in the prefrontal cortex, caudate nucleus and mediodorsal thalamic nucleus during delayed response performance of immature and adult rhesus monkeys. *Society for Neuroscience Abstracts* 6:86.

American Psychiatric Association. 1987. *Diagnostic and Statistical Manual of Mental Disorders.* 3rd ed., rev. Washington, D.C.

Anthony, J. C., L. LeResche, U. Niaz, M. R. Von Korff, and M. F. Folstein. 1982. Limits of the 'mini-mental state' as a screening test for dementia and delirium among hospital patients. *Psychological Medicine* 12:397–408.

Antonarakis, S. E., H. Youssoufian, and H. H. Kazazian, Jr. 1987. Molecular genetics of hemophilia A in man (factor VIII deficiency). *Molecular Biology and Medicine* 4:81–94.

Avila-Giron, R. 1973. Medical and social aspects of Huntington's chorea in the state of Zulia, Venezuela. *Advances in Neurology* 1:261–66.

Bamford, K., E. Caine, D. Kido, M. Harder, J. Kennedy, J. Behr, D. Goldblatt, C. Miller, R. Kurlan, and I. Shoulson. 1986. Neuropsychological impairment in early HD: Functional and CT correlates. *Neurology* 36 (suppl. 1):102–3.

Baraitser, M., J. Burn, and T. A. Fazzone. 1983. Huntington's chorea arising as a fresh mutation. *Journal of Medical Genetics* 20:459–75.

225

Barbeau, A., and J. R. Brunette. 1969. *Progress in Neurogenetics*. Pp. 666–73. Amsterdam: Excerpta Medical Foundation.

Barbeau, A., T. N. Chase, and G. W. Paulson, eds. 1973. Huntington's chorea, 1872–1972. *Advances in Neurology*. Vol. 1. New York: Raven Press.

Barczak, P., A. Pedler, S. Hunter, and T. Betts. 1987. Institutional care for patients with Huntington's chorea: Is there a better alternative? *Bulletin of the Royal College of Psychiatrists* 11:187–88.

Barr, A. N., J. H. Fischer, W. C. Koller, A. L. Spunt, and A. Singhal. 1988. Serum haloperidol concentration and choreiform movements in Huntington's disease. *Neurology* 38:84–88.

Bassi, S., M. G. Albizzati, G. U. Corsini, L. Frattola, R. Piolti, I. Suchy, and M. Trabucchi. 1986. Therapeutic experience with transdihydrolisuride in Huntington's disease. *Neurology* 36:984–86.

Beal, M. F., N. W. Kowall, D. W. Ellison, M. F. Mazurek, K. J. Swartz, and J. B. Martin. 1986. Replication of the neurochemical characteristics of Huntington's disease by quinolinic acid. *Nature* 321:168–71.

Beckman, L., B. Cedergren, B. Mattsson, and J. O. Ottosson. 1973. Genetic linkage in Huntington's chorea. *Advances in Neurology* 1:209–10.

Bell, J. 1934. Huntington's chorea. In *The Treasury of Human Genetics*. Vol. 4:1–29. Edited by R. A. Fischer. London: Cambridge University Press.

Bickford, J. A. R., and R. M. Ellison. 1953. High incidence of Huntington's chorea in the Duchy of Cornwall. *Journal of Mental Science* 99:291–94.

Bird, E. D., A. J. Caro, and J. B. Pilling. 1974. A sex related factor in the inheritance of Huntington's chorea. *Annals of Human Genetics* (London) 37:255–60.

Bird, E. D., J. Hewitt, P. M. Conneally, and M. R. Hayden. 1986. Linkage of the G8 marker on chromosome 4 to Huntington's disease in a large American black family. Letter in *New England Journal of Medicine* 315:1165–66.

Bittenbender, J. B., and F. A. Quadfasel. 1962. Rigid and akinetic forms of Huntington's chorea. *Archives of Neurology* 7:37–50.

Boehnke, M., P. M. Conneally, and K. Lange. 1983. Two models for a maternal factor in the inheritance of Huntington disease. *American Journal of Human Genetics* 35:845–60.

Bolt, J. M. W. 1970. Huntington's chorea in the west of Scotland. *British Journal of Psychiatry* 116:259–70.

Borkowski, J. G., A. L. Benton, and O. Spreen. 1967. Word fluency and brain damage. *Neuropsychologia* 5:135–40.

Brandt, J. 1985. Access to the knowledge in the dementia of Huntington's disease. *Developmental Neuropsychology* 1:335–48.

Brandt, J., and N. Butters. 1986. The neuropsychology of Huntington's disease. *Trends in Neuroscience* 9:118–20.

Brandt, J., S. E. Folstein, and M. F. Folstein. 1988. Differential cognitive impairment in Alzheimer's disease and Huntington's disease. *Annals of Neurology* 23:555–61.

Brandt, J., K. A. Quaid, S. E. Folstein, M. H. Abbott, M. L. Franz, P. R. Slavney, N. E. Maestri, P. B. Garber, L. M. Kasch, and H. H. Kazazian Jr. 1988. Presymptomatic testing for Huntington's disease with linked DNA markers: Clinical correlates. *American Journal of Human Genetics* 43 (abstract):311.

Brandt, J., M. E. Strauss, J. Larus, B. Jensen, S. E. Folstein, and M. F. Folstein. 1984.

Clinical correlates of dementia and disability in Huntington's disease. *Journal of Clinical Neuropsychology* 6:401–12.

Brothers, C. R. D. 1949. The history and incidence of Huntington's chorea in Tasmania. *Proceedings of the Royal Australian College of Physicians* 4:48–50.

Brothers, C. R. D. 1964. Huntington's chorea in Victoria and Tasmania. *Journal of the Neurological Sciences* 1:405–20.

Brothers, C. R. D., and Meadows, A. W. 1955. An investigation of Huntington's chorea in Victoria. *Journal of Mental Science* 101:548–63.

Brouwers, P., C. Cox, A. Martin, T. Chase, and P. Fedio. 1984. Differential perceptual-spatial impairment in Huntington's and Alzheimer's dementias. *Archives of Neurology* 41:1073–76.

Bruyn, G. W. 1968. Huntington's chorea: Historical, clinical and laboratory synopsis. In *Diseases of the Basal Ganglia*. Pp. 298–378. Edited by P. J. Vinken, and G. W. Bruyn. Amsterdam: North-Holland Publishing Company.

Bruyn, G. W. 1986. Chorea-acanthocytosis. In *Handbook of Clinical Neurology*. Vol. 49, 327–34. Edited by P. J. Vinken, G. W. Bruyn, and H. L. Klawans. New York: Elsevier Science Publishers.

Bruyn, G. W., and L. N. Went. 1986. Huntington's chorea. In *Handbook of Clinical Neurology*. Vol. 5(49), 267–77. Edited by P. J. Vinken, G. W. Bruyn, and H. L. Klawans. New York: Elsevier Science Publishers.

Burns, A., S. E. Folstein, J. Brandt, and M. F. Folstein. (In preparation). Clinical assessment of irritability, aggression, and apathy in Huntington's and Alzheimer's disease.

Buschke, H. 1973. Selective reminding for analysis of memory and learning. *Journal of Verbal Learning and Verbal Behavior* 12:543–50.

Butters, N. 1984. The clinical aspects of memory disorders: Contributions from experimental studies of amnesia and dementia. *Journal of Clinical Neuropsychology* 6:17–36.

Butters, N., D. Sax, K. Montgomery, and S. Tarlow. 1978. Comparison of the neuropsychological deficits associated with early and advanced Huntington's disease. *Archives of Neurology* 35:585–89.

Butters, N., S. Tarlow, L. S. Cermak, and D. Sachs. 1976. A comparison of the information processing deficits of patients with Huntington's chorea and Korsakoff's syndrome. *Cortex* 12:134–44.

Butters, N., J. Wolfe, and E. Granholm. 1986. An assessment of verbal recall, recognition and fluency abilities in patients with Huntington's disease. *Cortex* 22:11–32.

Caine, E. D., K. A. Bamford, R. B. Schiffer, I. Shoulson, and S. Levy. 1986. A controlled neuropsychological comparison of Huntington's disease and multiple sclerosis. *Archives of Neurology* 43:249–54.

Caine, E. D., M. H. Ebert, and H. Weingartner. 1977. An outline for the analysis of dementia: The memory disorder of Huntington disease. *Neurology* 27:1087–92.

Caine, E. D., R. D. Hunt, H. Weingartner, and M. H. Ebert. 1978. Huntington's dementia: Clinical and neuropsychological features. *Archives of General Psychiatry* 35:377–84.

Calne, D. B., and W. R. W. Martin. 1986. Chemistry of the basal ganglia. In *Handbook of Clinical Neurology*. Vol. 49, 33–46. Edited by P. J. Vinken, G. W. Bruyn, and H. L. Klawans. New York: Elsevier Science Publishers.

Carpenter, M. B. 1986. Anatomy of the basal ganglia. In *Handbook of Clinical Neurology*. Vol. 49, 1–18. Edited by P. J. Vinken, G. W. Bruyn, and H. L. Klawans. New York: Elsevier Science Publishers.

Carpenter, M. B., J. R. Whittier, and F. A. Mettler. 1950. Analysis of choreoid hyperkinesia in the rhesus monkey: Surgical and pharmacological analysis of hyperkinesia resulting from lesions in the subthalamic nucleus of Luys. *Journal of Comparative Neurology* 92:293–331.

Carrasco, L. H., and C. S. Mukherji. 1986. Atrophy of corpus striatum in normal male at risk of Huntington's chorea. *Lancet* 14(June):1388–89.

Chandler, J. H., T. E. Reed, and R. N. DeJong. 1960. Huntington's chorea in Michigan: III. Clinical observations. *Neurology* 10:148–53.

Chase, G. A., L. E. Markson, R. Brookmeyer, and S. E. Folstein. 1986. Covariate-dependent genetic counseling in Huntington's disease. *Journal of Neurogenetics* 3:215–23.

Chase, T. N., N. S. Wexler, and A. Barbeau, eds. 1979. Huntington's disease. In *Advances in Neurology*. Vol. 23. New York: Raven Press.

Chiu, E., and C. J. Brackenridge. 1976. A probable cause of mutation in Huntington's disease. *Journal of Medical Genetics* 13:75–77.

Choi, W. D. 1988. Glutamate neurotoxicity and diseases of the nervous system. *Neuron* 1:623–34.

Conneally, P. M. 1984. Huntington disease: Genetics and epidemiology. *American Journal of Human Genetics* 36:506–26.

Cotman, C. W., D. T. Monaghan, O. P. Ottersen, and J. Strom-Mathisen. 1987. Anatomical organization or excitatory amino acid receptors and their pathways. *Trends in Neuroscience* 10:273–79.

Coyle, J. T., and R. Schwarcz. 1976. Lesions of striatal neurones with kainic acid provides a model for Huntington's chorea. *Nature* 263:244–46.

Crane, G. E. 1973. Tardive dyskinesia and Huntington's chorea: Drug induced and heredity dyskinesia. *Advances in Neurology* 1:115–22.

Critchley, M. 1973. Great Britain and the early history of Huntington's chorea. *Advances in Neurology* 1:13–17.

Cross, A. J., P. Slater, and G. P. Reynolds. 1986. Reduced high-affinity glutamate uptake sites in the brains of patients with Huntington's disease. *Neuroscience Letters* 67:199–202.

Davenport, C. B., and E. B. Muncey. 1916. Huntington's chorea in relation to heredity and eugenics. *American Journal of Insanity* 73:195–222.

David, A. S., D. V. Jeste, M. F. Folstein, and S. E. Folstein. 1987. Voluntary movement dysfunction in Huntington's disease and tardive dyskinesia. *Acta Neurologica Scandinavia* 75:130–39.

Deckel, A. W., R. G. Robinson, J. T. Coyle, and P. R. Sanberg. 1983. Reversal of long-term locomotor abnormalities in the kainic acid model of Huntington's disease by day 18 fetal striatal implants. *European Journal of Pharmacology* 93:287–88.

DeJong, R. N. 1973. The history of Huntington's chorea in the United States of America. *Advances in Neurology* 1:19–27.

DeLong, M. J., T. H. Murphy, M. Miyamoto, and J. T. Coyle. 1988. *Society for Neuroscience Abstracts* 14:168.20, p. 420.

DeLong, M. R., and A. P. Georgopoulos. 1979. Motor functions of the basal ganglia as revealed by studies of single unit activities in the behaving primate. *Advances in Neurology* 24:131–40.

Derogotis, L. 1983. *SCL-90R Manual-II*. Towson: Clinical Psychometric Research.

Deroover, J., F. Baro, R. P. Bourguignon, and P. Smets. 1984. Tiapride versus placebo: A double-blind comparative study in the management of Huntington's chorea. *Current Medical Research and Opinion* 9:329–38.

De Souza, E. B., P. J. Whitehouse, S. E. Folstein, D. L. Price, and W. W. Vale. 1988. Corticotropin-releasing hormone (CRH) is decreased in the basal ganglia in Huntington's disease. *Brain Research* (Short Communications BRE 22639).

DeVeaugh-Geiss, J., ed. 1982. *Tardive Dyskinesia and Related Involuntary Movement Disorders*. Boston: John Wright, PSG, Inc.

Dewhurst, K. 1970. Personality disorder in Huntington's disease. *Psychiatric Clinica* 3:221–29.

Dewhurst, K., J. E. Oliver, and A. L. McKnight. 1970. Socio-psychiatric consequences of Huntington's disease. *British Journal of Psychiatry* 116:255–58.

Dewhurst, K., J. E. Oliver, K. L. K. Trick, and A. L. McKnight. 1969. Neuropsychiatric aspects of Huntington's disease. *Confinia Neurologica* 31:258–68.

Diefendorf, A. R., ed. 1907. *Clinical Psychiatry: A Text-book for Students and Physicians*. New York: Macmillan Company.

DiFiglia, M. 1987. Synaptic organization of cholinergic neurons in the monkey neostriatum. *Journal of Comparative Neurology* 255:245–58.

DiFiglia, M., P. Pasik, and T. Pasik. 1976. A Golgi study of neuronal types in the neostriatum of monkeys. *Brain Research* 114:245–56.

DiFiglia, M., P. Pasik, and T. Pasik. 1982. A Golgi and ultrastructural study of the monkey globus pallidus. *Journal of Comparative Neurology* 212:53–75.

DiFiglia, M., T. Pasik, and P. Pasik. 1978. A Golgi study of afferent fibers in the neostriatum of monkeys. *Brain Research* 152:341–47.

DiFiglia, M., T. Pasik, and P. Pasik. 1980. Ultrastructure of Golgi-impregnated and gold-toned spiny and aspiny neurons in the monkey neostriatum. *Journal of Neurocytology* 9:471–92.

Divac, I., H. E. Rosvold, and M. K. Szwarcbart. 1967. Behavioral effects of selective ablation of the caudate nucleus. *Journal of Comparative and Physiological Psychology* 63:181–90.

Dodge, R., R. C. Travis, and J. C. Fox, Jr. 1930. Optic nystagmus III. Characteristics of the slow phase. *Archives of Neurology and Psychiatry, Chicago* 24:21–34.

Dohrenwend, B. S., L. Krasnoff, A. R. Askenasy, and B. P. Dohrenwend. 1982. *Handbook of Stress*. Edited by L. Goldberger and S. Breznitz. New York: The Free Press.

Dom, R., M. Malfroid, and F. Baro. 1976. Neuropathology of Huntington's chorea. *Neurology* 26:64–68.

Enna, S. J., J. P. Bennett, Jr., D. B. Bylund, S. H. Snyder, E. D. Bird, and L. L. Iversen. 1976. Alterations of brain neurotransmitter receptor binding in Huntington's chorea. *Brain Research* 116:531–37.

Farrer, L. A., and P. M. Conneally. 1985. A genetic model for age at onset in Huntington disease. *American Journal of Human Genetics* 37:350–57.

Farrer, L. A., P. M. Conneally, and P. I. Yu. 1984. The natural history of Huntington's disease: Possible roles of "aging genes." *American Journal of Medical Genetics* 18:115–23.

Faught, E., J. C. Falgout, and D. A. Leli. 1983. Late-onset variant of Huntington's chorea. *Southern Medical Journal* 76:1266–70.

Fedio, P., C. S. Cox, A. Neophytides, G. Canal-Frederick, and T. N. Chase. 1979. Neuropsychological profile of Huntington's disease: Patients and those at risk. *Advances in Neurology* 23:239–55.

Feigenbaum, L. A., A. M. Graybiel, J. P. Vonsattel, E. P. Richardson, Jr., and E. D. Bird. 1986. Striasomal markers in the striatum in Huntington's disease. *Society for Neuroscience Abstracts* 12.

Ferrante, R. J., N. W. Kowall, M. F. Beal, J. B. Martin, E. D. Bird, and E. P. Richardson, Jr. 1987. Morphologic and histochemical characteristics of a spared subset of striatal neurons in Huntington's disease. *Journal of Neuropathology and Experimental Neurology* 46:12–27.

Ferrante, R. J., N. W. Kowall, E. P. Richardson, Jr., E. D. Bird, and J. B. Martin. 1986. Topography of enkephalin, substance P and acetylcholinesterase staining in Huntington's disease striatum. *Neuroscience Letters* 71:283–88.

Fisher, J. M., J. L. Kennedy, E. D. Caine, and I. Shoulson. 1983. Dementia in Huntington disease: A cross-sectional analysis of intellectual decline. In *The Dementias*, edited by R. Mayeux, and W. G. Rosen. Pp. 229–38. New York: Raven Press.

Fog, R., and H. Pakkenberg. 1980. Combination treatment of choreiform and dyskinetic syndromes with tetrabenazine and pimozide. In *Tardive Dyskinesia*, edited by W. E. Fann, R. C. Smith, J. M. Davis, and E. F. Domino. Pp. 507–10. New York: Spectrum.

Folstein, M. F., S. E. Folstein, and P. R. McHugh. 1975. "Mini-Mental State": A practical method for grading the cognitive state of patients for the clinician. *Journal of Psychiatric Research* 2:189–98.

Folstein, M. F., R. Robinson, S. Folstein, and P. R. McHugh. 1985. Depression and neurological disorders: New treatment opportunities for elderly depressed patients. *Journal of Affective Disorders* (suppl. 1): S11–14.

Folstein, S. E., M. H. Abbott, G. A. Chase, B. A. Jensen, and M. F. Folstein. 1983. The association of affective disorder with Huntington's disease in a case series and in families. *Psychological Medicine* 13:537–42.

Folstein, S. E., M. H. Abbott, M. L. Franz, S. Huang, G. A. Chase, and M. F. Folstein. 1984. Phenotypic heterogeneity in Huntington disease. *Journal of Neurogenetics* 1:175–84.

Folstein, S. E., M. Abbott, R. Moser, I. Parhad, A. Clark, and M. Folstein. 1981. A phenocopy of Huntington's disease: Lacunar infarcts of the corpus striatum. *Johns Hopkins Medical Journal* 148:104–13.

Folstein, S. E., G. A. Chase, W. E. Wahl, A. M. McDonnell, and M. F. Folstein. 1987. Huntington disease in Maryland: Clinical aspects of racial variation. *American Journal of Human Genetics* 41:168–79.

Folstein, S. E., and M. F. Folstein. 1987. Diseases of the caudate as a model for a manic depressive disorder. In *An International Conference on the Basal Ganglia (Abstracts)*. The University of Leeds.

Folstein, S. E., M. F. Folstein, and P. R. McHugh. 1979. Psychiatric syndromes in Huntington's disease. *Advances in Neurology* 23:281–89.

Folstein, S. E., M. L. Franz, B. Jensen, G. A. Chase, and M. F. Folstein. 1983. Conduct disorder and affective disorder among the offspring of patients with Huntington's disease. In *Childhood Psychopathology and Development*, edited by S. B. Guze, F. J. Earls, and J. E. Barrett. Pp. 231–45. New York: Raven Press.

Folstein, S. E., B. Jensen, R. J. Leigh, and M. F. Folstein. 1983. The measurement of abnormal movement: Methods developed for Huntington's disease. *Neurobehavioral Toxicology and Teratology* 5:605–9.

Folstein, S. E., R. J. Leigh, I. M. Parhad, and M. F. Folstein. 1986. The diagnosis of Huntington's disease. *Neurology* 36:1279–83.

Folstein, S. E., J. A. Phillips III, D. A. Meyers, G. A. Chase, M. H. Abbott, M. L. Franz, P. G. Waber, H. H. Kazazian Jr., P. M. Conneally, W. Hobbs, R. Tanzi, A. Faryniarz, K. Gibbons, and J. Gusella. 1985. Huntington's disease: Two families with differing clinical features show linkage to the G8 probe. *Science* 229:776–79.

Ford, M. F. 1986. Treatment of depression in Huntington's disease with monoamine oxidase inhibitors. *British Journal of Psychiatry* 149:654–56.

Foster, N. L., T. N. Chase, A. Denaro, T. A. Hare, and C. A. Tamminga. 1983. THIP treatment of Huntington's disease. *Neurology* (Cleveland) 33:637–39.

Freinhar, J. P., W. A. Alvarez, and M. L. Chambers. 1985. Combination psychopharmacological and behavioral therapy in Huntington's chorea: A case study. *International Journal of Psychosomatics* 32:17–19.

Fuster, J. M., and G. E. Alexander. 1973. Firing changes in cells of the nucleus medialis dorsalis associated with delayed response behavior. *Brain Research* 61:79–91.

Garron, D. C. 1973. Huntington's chorea and schizophrenia. *Advances in Neurology* 1:729–34.

Gebbink, T. B. 1968. Huntington's chorea: Fibre changes in the basal ganglia. In *Handbook of Clinical Neurology*. Vol. 6, 399–408. Edited by P. J. Vinken, and G. W. Bruyn. New York: American Elsevier Publishers.

Gerfen, C. R. 1984. The neostriatal mosaic: Compartmentalization of corticostriatal input and striatonigral output systems. *Nature* 311:461–64.

Gerfen, C. R. 1986. The developmental and biochemical basis of dual "patch" and "matrix" nigrostriatal dopaminergic systems in the rat. *Neuroscience Abstracts* A362.8, p. 1327.

Gerfen, C. R., K. G. Baimbridge, and J. Thibault. 1987. The neostriatal mosaic: III. Biochemical and developmental dissociation of patch-matrix mesostriatal systems. *Journal of Neuroscience* 7:3935–44.

Gerfen, C. R., M. Herkenham, and J. Thibault. 1987. The neostriatal mosaic: II. Patch- and matrix-directed mesostriatal dopaminergic and non-dopaminergic systems. *Journal of Neuroscience* 7:3915–34.

Geshwind, N. 1965. Disconnexion syndromes in animals and man. *Brain* 88:237–94, 585–44.

Gilliam, T. C., M. Bucan, M. E. MacDonald, M. Zimmer, J. L. Haines, S. V. Cheng, T. M. Pohl, R. H. Meyers, W. L. Whaley, B. A. Allitto, A. Faryniarz, J. J. Wasmuth, A. M. Frischauf, P. M. Conneally, H. Lehrach, and J. F. Gusella. 1987. A DNA segment encoding two genes very tightly linked to Huntington's disease. *Science* 238:950–52.

Gilliam, T. C., R. E. Tanzi, J. L. Haines, T. I. Bonner, A. G. Faryniarz, W. J. Hobbs, M. E. MacDonald, S. V. Cheng, S. E. Folstein, P. M. Conneally, N. S. Wexler, and J. F. Gusella. 1987. Localization of the Huntington's disease gene to a small segment of chromosome 4 flanked by D4S10 and the telomere. *Cell* 50:565–71.

Gordon, W. P., and J. Illes. 1987. Neurolinguistic characteristics of language production in Huntington's disease: A preliminary report. *Brain and Language* 31:1–10.

Graveland, G. A., R. S. Williams, and M. DiFiglia. 1985a. A Golgi study of the human neostriatum: Neurons and afferent fibers. *Journal of Comparative Neurology* 234:317–33.

Graveland, G. A., R. S. Williams, and M. DiFiglia. 1985b. Evidence for degenerative and regenerative changes in neostriatal spiny neurons in Huntington's disease. *Science* 227:770–73.

Graybiel, A. M. 1984. Neurochemically specified subsystems in the basal ganglia. In *Functions of the Basal Ganglia*, edited by D. Evered. Pp. 114–49. Ciba Foundations Symposium 107. London: Pitman.

Graybiel, A. M. 1986. Neuropeptides in the basal ganglia. In *Neuropeptides in Neurologic and Psychiatric Disease*, edited by J. B. Martin, and J. D. Barchas. Pp. 135–61. New York: Raven Press.

Graybiel, A. M., R. W. Baughman, and F. Eckenstein. 1986. Cholinergic neuropil of the striatum observes striosomal boundaries. *Nature* 323:625–27.

Graybiel, A. M., and C. W. Ragsdale, Jr. 1978. Histochemically distinct compartments in the striatum of human, monkey, and cat demonstrated by acetylthiocholinesterase staining. *Proceedings of the National Academy of Sciences of the United States of America* 75:5723–26.

Graybiel, A. M., and C. W. Ragsdale, Jr. 1979. Fiber connections of the basal ganglia. In *Development and Chemical Specificity of Neurons*, edited by M. Cuenod, G. W. Kreutzberg, and F. E. Bloom. Pp. 239–83. Amsterdam: Elsevier Science Publishers.

Graybiel, A. M., and C. W. Ragsdale, Jr. 1983. Biochemical anatomy of the striatum. In *Chemical Neuroanatomy*, edited by P. C. Emson. Pp. 427–504. New York: Raven Press.

Green, J. B., E. S. Dickenson, and J. R. Gunderman. 1973. Epilepsy in Huntington's chorea: Clinical and neurophysiological studies. *Advances in Neurology* 1:105–13.

Gusella, J., N. S. Wexler, P. M. Conneally, S. L. Naylor, M. A. Anderson, R. E. Tanzi, P. C. Watkins, K. Ottina, M. R. Wallace, A. Y. Sakaguchi, A. B. Young, I. Shoulson, E. Bonilla, and J. B. Martin. 1983. A polymorphic DNA marker genetically linked to Huntington's disease. *Nature* 306:234–38.

Haines, J., R. Tanzi, N. Wexler, P. Harper, S. Folstein, J. Cassiman, R. Meyers, A. Young, M. Hayden, A. Falek, E. Tolosa, S. Crespi, G. Campanella, G. Holmgren, M. Anvret, I. Kanazawa, J. Gusella, and M. Conneally. 1986. No evidence of linkage heterogeneity between Huntington's disease (HD) and G8 (D4S10). *American Journal of Human Genetics* 39:A156.

Hamada, I., and M. R. DeLong. 1988. Lesions of the primate subthalamic nucleus (STN) reduce tonic and phasic neural activity in globus pallidus. *Society for Neuroscience Abstract* 14:719.

Hamilton, A. S. 1908. A report of twenty-seven cases of chronic progressive chorea. *American Journal of Insanity* 64:28, 404–75.

Hans, M. B., and T. H. Gilmore. 1968. Social aspects of Huntington's chorea. *British Journal of Psychiatry* 114:93–98.

Hans, M. B., and A. H. Koeppen. 1980. Huntington's chorea: Its impact on the spouse. *Journal of Nervous and Mental Disease* 168:209–14.

Hanssen, O. 1914. Den saetesdalske chorea St. Viti. *Medicinsk Revew* (Bergen) 31:569–79.

Harper, P. S., and M. Sarfarazi. 1985. Genetic prediction and family structure in Huntington's chorea. *British Medical Journal* 290:1929–31.

Harper, P. S., A. Tyler, S. Smith, P. Jones, R. G. Newcombe, and V. McBroom. 1982. A genetic register for Huntington's chorea in South Wales. *Journal of Medical Genetics* 19:241–45.

Harper, P. S., D. A. Walker, A. Tyler, R. G. Newcombe, and K. Davies. 1979. Huntington's chorea: The basis for long-term prevention. *Lancet* 2:346–49.

Harper, P. S., S. Youngman, M. A. Anderson, M. Sarfarazi, O. Quarrell, R. Tanzi, D. Shaw, P. Wallace, P. M. Conneally, and J. F. Gusella. 1985. Genetic linkage between Huntington's disease and the DNA polymorphism G8 in south Wales families. *Journal of Medical Genetics* 22:447–50.

Hawkins, M. R., E. A. Murphy, and H. Abbey. 1965. The familial component in longevity. *Bulletin of the Johns Hopkins Hospital* 117:24–36.

Hayden, M. R. 1979. Huntington's chorea in South Africa. Ph.D. dissertation, University of South Africa.

Hayden, M. R., ed. 1981. *Huntington's Chorea*. Berlin: Springer-Verlag.

Hayden, M. R., and P. Beighton. 1977. Huntington's chorea in the cape coloured community of South Africa. *South African Medical Journal* 52:886–88.

Hayden, M. R., J. M. MacGregor, and P. H. Beighton. 1980. The prevalence of Huntington's chorea in South Africa. *South African Medical Journal* 58:193–96.

Hayden, M. R., J. M. MacGregor, D. S. Saffer, and P. H. Beighton. 1982. The high frequency of juvenile Huntington's chorea in South Africa. *Journal of Medical Genetics* 19:94–97.

Hayden, M. R., W. R. W. Martin, A. J. Stoessl, C. Clark, S. Hollenberg, M. J. Adam, W. Ammann, R. Harrop, J. Rogers, T. Ruth, C. Sayre, and B. D. Pate. 1986. Positron emission tomography in the early diagnosis of Huntington's disease. *Neurology* 36:888–94.

Hayden, M. R., J. A. Soles, and R. H. Ward. 1985. Age of onset in siblings of persons with juvenile Huntington disease. *Clinical Genetics* 28:100–105.

Hayden, M. R., S. Youngman, J. Hewitt, D. Allard, M. Altherr, C. Robbins, J. Haines, P. S. Harper, C. Collins, C. Payne, A. Roses, M. Pericak-Vance, B. Smith, J. Wasmuth. 1988. The gene causing Huntington disease is telomeric to a variable number of tandem repeat (VNTR) polymorphism detected by D4S95 and a new DNA marker D4S90. *American Journal of Human Genetics* 43:abstract 342.

Heathfield, K. W. G. 1967. Huntington's chorea: Investigation into the prevalence of this disease in the area covered by the North East Metropolitan Regional Hospital Board. *Brain* 90:203–32.

Heathfield, K. W. G., and I. C. MacKenzie. 1971. Huntington's chorea in Bedfordshire, England. *Guy's Hospital Report* 120:295–309.

Heimer, L., and R. D. Wilson. 1975. The subcortical projections of the allocortex: Similarities in the neural associations of the hippocampus, the piriform cortex, and the neocortex. In *Golgi Centennial Symposium: Perspectives in Neurobiology*, edited by M. Santini. Pp. 177–93. New York: Raven Press.

Hughes, E. M. 1924. Social significance of Huntington's chorea. *American Journal of Psychiatry* 4:537–74.

Huntington, G. 1872. On chorea. *Advances in Neurology* 1:33–35.

Jankovic, J. 1986. Myoglobinuric renal failure in Huntington's chorea. *Neurology* 36:138–49.

Jelgersma, G. 1908. Neue pathologische Befunde bei Paralysis agitans und bei chronischer Chorea. *Neurol. Zbl.* 27:995.

Jeste, D. V., L. Barban, and J. Parisi. 1984. Reduced Purkinje cell density in Huntington's disease. *Experimental Neurology* 85:78–86.

Jones, M. B., and C. R. Phillips. 1970. Affected parent and age of onset in Huntington's chorea. *Journal of Medical Genetics* 7:20–21.

Jongen, P. J. H., W. O. Renier, and F. J. M. Gabreels. 1980. Seven cases of Huntington's disease in childhood and levodopa induced improvement in the hypokinetic-rigid form. *Clinical Neurology and Neurosurgery* 82:251–61.

Jorgenson, R. J., F. E. Yoder, and S. D. Shapiro. 1980. *The Pedigree: A Basic Guide*. Charleston: The Grendel Company.

Josiassen, R. C., L. M. Curry, and E. L. Mancall. 1983. Development of neuropsychological deficits in Huntington's disease. *Archives of Neurology* 40:791–96.

Josiassen, R. C., L. Curry, R. A. Roemer, and C. DeBease. 1982. Patterns of intellectual deficit in Huntington's disease. *Journal of Clinical Neuropsychology* 4:173–83.

Kereshi, S., R. E. Schlagenhauff, and K. S. Richardson. 1980. Myoclonic and major seizures in early adult Huntington's chorea: Case-report and electro-clinical findings. *Clinical Electroencephalography* 11:44–47.

King, M. 1985. Alcohol abuse in Huntington's disease. *Psychological Medicine* 15:815–19.

Kita, H., and S. T. Kitai. 1987. Efferent projections of the subthalamic nucleus in the rat: Light and electron microscopic analysis with the PHA-L method. *Journal of Comparative Neurology* 260:435–52.

Klein, J. 1980. *Woodie Guthrie: A Life*. New York: Alfred A. Knopf, Inc.

Koller, W. C., and J. Trimble. 1985. The gait abnormality of Huntington's disease. *Neurology* 35:1450–54.

Kosky, R. 1981. Children and Huntington's disease: Some clinical observations of children at-risk. *Medical Journal of Australia* 1:405–7.

Koroshetz, W. J., R. H. Meyers, C. Mastromauro, and J. B. Martin. 1988. Presymptomatic testing for Huntington's disease. *Neurology* 38:360, abstract 7.

Kozachuk, W., V. Salanga, J. Conomy, and A. Smith. 1986. MRI (Magnetic Resonance Imaging) in Huntington's disease. *Neurology* (suppl. 1) 36:310.

Kramer, J. H., D. C. Delis, M. J. Blusewicz, J. Brandt, B. A. Ober, and M. Strauss. 1988. Verbal memory errors in Alzheimer's and Huntington's dementias. *Developmental Neuropsychology* 4:1–15.

Krush, A. J., and K. A. Evans, eds. 1984. *Family Studies in Genetic Disorders*. Springfield, Ill.: Charles C Thomas Publisher.

Kuhl, D. E., C. H. Markham, E. J. Metter, W. H. Riege, M. E. Phelps, and J. C. Mazziotta. 1985. Local cerebral glucose utilization in symptomatic and presymptomatic Huntington's disease. In *Brain Imaging and Brain Function*, edited by L. Sokoloff. Pp. 199–209. New York: Raven Press.

Kuhl, D. E., M. E. Phelps, C. H. Markham, E. J. Metter, W. H. Riege, and J. Winter. 1982. Cerebral metabolism and atrophy in Huntington's disease determined by [18]FDG and computed tomographic scan. *Annals of Neurology* 12:425–34.

Lange, H., G. Thorner, A. Hopf, and K. F. Schroder. 1976. Morphometric studies of the neuropathological changes in choreatic diseases. *Journal of the Neurological Sciences* 28:401–25.

Lasker, A. G., D. S. Zee, T. C. Hain, S. E. Folstein, and H. S. Singer. 1987. Saccades in Huntington's disease: Initiation defects and distractibility. *Neurology* 37:427–31.

Lasker, A. G., D. S. Zee, T. C. Hain, S. E. Folstein, and H. S. Singer. 1988. Saccades in Huntington's disease: Slowing and dysmetria. *Neurology* 38:364–70.

Leigh, R. J., S. A. Newman, S. E. Folstein, A. G. Lasker, and B. A. Jensen. 1983. Abnormal ocular motor control in Huntington's disease. *Neurology* (Cleveland) 33:1268–75.

Leonard, D. P., M. A. Kidson, P. J. Shannon, and J. Brown. 1974. Double blind trial of lithium carbonate and haloperidol in Huntington's chorea. *Lancet* (November 16), 1208–9.

Leopold, N. A., and M. C. Kagel. 1985. Dysphagia in Huntington's disease. *Archives of Neurology* 42:57–60.

Lilienfeld, A. M., and D. E. Lilienfeld. 1980. *Foundations of Epidemiology*. 2nd ed. New York: Oxford University Press.

Lindstrom, J. A., W. B. Bias, R. N. Schimke, D. K. Ziegler, M. L. Rivas, G. A. Chase, and V. A. McKusick. 1973. Genetic linkage in Huntington's chorea. *Advances in Neurology* 1:203–8.

Lipton, R. B., D. L. Levy, P. S. Holzman, and S. Levin. 1983. Eye movement dysfunctions in psychiatric patients: A review. *Schizophrenia Bulletin* 9:13–32.

London, E. D., H. I. Yamamura, E. D. Bird, and J. T. Coyle. 1981. Decreased receptor-binding sites for kainic acid in brains of patients with Huntington's disease. *Biological Psychiatry* 16:155–62.

Lucas, D. R., and J. P. Newhouse. 1957. The toxic effect of sodium L-glutamate on the inner layers of the retina. A.M.A. *Archives of Opththalmology* 58:193–201.

Lugaresi, E., F. Cirignotta, and P. Montagna. 1986. Nocturnal paroxysmal dystonia. *Journal of Neurology, Neurosurgery and Psychiatry* 49:375–80.

Lund, J. C. 1860. 'Chorea Sancti Viti i Satesdalen' Beretning om Sundhedstilstanden og medicinalforholdene i. *Norge* i, p. 137.

Lyle, O. E., and I. I. Gottesman. 1977. Premorbid psychometric indicators of the gene for Huntington's disease. *Journal of Consulting and Clinical Psychology* 45:1011–22.

Lyle, O. E., and I. I. Gottesman. 1979. Subtle cognitive deficits as 15- to 20-year precursors of Huntington's disease. *Advances in Neurology* 23:227–38.

Lyon, R. L. 1962. Huntington's chorea in the Moray Firth area. *British Medical Journal* 12 (May): 1301–6.

Machlin, L. J., and A. Bendich. 1987. Free radical tissue damage: Protective role of antioxidant nutrients. *Federation of American Societies for Experimental Biology* 1:441–45.

Maestri, N. E., T. H. Beaty, S. E. Folstein, and D. A. Meyers. 1987. Use of the G8 probe in predicting risk of Huntington disease. *American Journal of Human Genetics* 28:989–97.

Malach, R., and A. M. Graybiel. 1986. Mosaic architecture of the somatic sensory-recipient sector of the cat's striatum. *Journal of Neuroscience* 6:3436–58.

Marsden, C. D. 1984. The pathophysiology of movement disorders. In *Neurologic Clinics: Symposium of Movement Disorders* 2:435–59.

Martindale, B., and V. Bottomley. 1980. The management of families with Huntington's chorea: A case study to illustrate some recommendations. *Journal of Child Psychiatry and Psychology* 21:343–51.

Martone, M., N. Butters, M. Payne, J. T. Becker, and D. S. Sax. 1984. Dissociations between skill learning and verbal recognition in amnesia and dementia. *Archives of Neurology* 41:965–70.

Marx, R. N. 1973. Huntington's chorea in Minnesota. *Advances in Neurology* 1:237–43.

Mattsson, B. 1973. Huntington's chorea and lithium therapy. *Lancet* 31 (March):718–19.

Mattsson, B. 1974a. Huntington's chorea in Sweden: I. Prevalence and genetic data. *Acta Psychiatrica Scandinavica. Supplementum* 255:211–19.

Mattsson, B. 1974b. Huntington's chorea in Sweden: II. Social and clinical data. *Acta Psychiatrica Scandinavica Supplementum* 255:221–35.

May, P. C., and P. N. Gray. 1985. The mechanism of glutamate-induced degeneration of cultured Huntington's disease and control fibroblasts. *Journal of the Neurological Sciences* 70:101–12.

Mayeux, R., Y. Stern, A. Herman, L. Greenbaum, and S. Fahn. 1986. Correlates of early disability in Huntington's disease. *Annals of Neurology* 20:727–31.

Mayr, E. 1963. *Animal Species and Evolution.* Cambridge: Harvard University Press.

Mazziotta, J. C., M. E. Phelps, J. J. Pahl, S. C. Huang, L. R. Baxter, W. H. Riege, J. M. Hoffman, D. E. Kuhl, A. B. Lanto, J. A. Wapenski, and C. H. Markham. 1987. Reduced cerebral glucose metabolism in asymptomatic subjects at risk for Huntington's disease. *New England Journal of Medicine* 316:357–62.

McGeer, E. G., and P. L. McGeer. 1976. Duplication of biochemical changes of Huntington's chorea. In *Progress in Neurogenetics*, edited by A. Barbeau and T. R. Brunette. Pp. 645–50. Amsterdam: Excerpta Medica Foundation.

McHugh, P. R. 1987. The basal ganglia: The region, the integration of its systems and implications for psychiatry and neurology. Proceedings of the University of Leeds International Conference on the Basal Ganglia.

McHugh, P. R., and M. F. Folstein. 1973. Subcortical dementia. Address to the American Academy of Neurology, April, Boston, MA.

McHugh, P. R., and M. F. Folstein. 1975. Psychiatric syndromes of Huntington's chorea: A clinical and phenomenologic study. In *Psychiatric Aspects of Neurologic Disease*, edited by D. F. Benson, and D. Blumer. New York: Grune & Stratton, Inc.

McKusick, V. A. 1986. *Mendelian Inheritance in Man.* 7th ed. Baltimore: Johns Hopkins University Press.

Meissen, G. J., R. H. Myers, C. A. Mastromauro, W. J. Koroshetz, K. W. Klinger, L. A. Farrer, P. A. Watkins, J. F. Gusella, E. D. Bird, and J. B. Martin. 1988. Predictive testing for Huntington's disease with use of a linked DNA marker. *New England Journal of Medicine* 318:535–42.

Merritt, A. D., P. M. Conneally, N. F. Rahman, and A. L. Drew. 1969. Juvenile Huntington's chorea. In *Progress in Neurogenetics*, edited by A. Barbeau and T. R. Brunette. Pp. 645–50. Amsterdam: Excerpta Medica Foundation.

Miller, E. 1976. The social work component in community-based action on behalf of victims of Huntington's disease. *Social Work in Health Care* 2:25–32.

Minski, L., and E. Guttman. 1938. Huntington's chorea: A study of thirty-four families. *Journal of Mental Science* 84:21–96.

Miyamoto, M., T. H. Murphy, R. L. Schnaar, and J. T. Coyle. 1988. Antioxidants protect against cytotoxicity in a neuronal cell line. *Society for Neuroscience* 14:168.19, p. 420.

Miyamoto, M. et al. submitted. Antioxidants protect against striatal glutamate damage in rats.

Mortimer, J. A., S.-P. Jun, M. A. Kuskowski, F. J. Pirozzolo, and D. D. Webster. 1987. Cognitive and behavioral disorders in Parkinson's disease. *An International Conference on the Basal Ganglia.* July 14–17. Abstract 14.15. The University of Leeds, England.

Moses, Jr., J. A., C. J. Golden, P. A. Berger, and A. M. Wisniewski. 1981. Neuropsychological deficits in early, middle, and late stage Huntington's disease as measured by the Luria-Nebraska neuropsychological battery. *International Journal of Neuroscience* 14:95–100.

Moss, M. B., M. S. Albert, N. Butters, and M. Payne. 1986. Differential patterns of memory loss among patients with Alzheimer's disease, Huntington's disease, and alcoholic Korsakoff's syndrome. *Archives of Neurology* 43:239–46.

Murphy, E. A. 1978. Genetic and evolutionary fitness. *American Journal of Medical Genetics* 2:51–79.

Murphy, E. A., A. J. Krush, M. Dietz, and C. A. Rohde. 1980. Heredity polyposis coli: III. Genetic and evolutionary fitness. *American Journal of Human Genetics* 32:700–713.

Murthy, G. G., A. D. Rosen, and M. Babu. 1977. Thyrotoxicosis with Huntington's chorea. *New York State Journal of Medicine* 77:1322–24.

Myers, R. H., D. Goldman, E. D. Bird, D. S. Sax, C. R. Merril, M. Schoenfeld, and P. A. Wolf. 1983. Maternal transmission in Huntington's disease. *Lancet*, 208–10.

Myers, R. H., J. J. Madden, J. L. Teague, and A. Falek. 1982. Factors related to onset age of Huntington disease. *American Journal of Human Genetics* 34:481–88.

Myers, R. H., D. S. Sax, M. Schoenfeld, E. D. Bird, P. A. Wolfe, J. P. Vonsattel, R. F. White, and J. B. Martin. 1985. Late onset of Huntington's disease. *Journal of Neurology, Neurosurgery, and Psychiatry* 48:530–34.

Myrianthopoulos, N. E. 1966. Huntington's chorea. *Journal of Medical Genetics* 3:298–314.

Narabayashi, H. 1973. Huntington's chorea in Japan: Review of the literature. *Advances in Neurology* 1:253–59.

Nathans, D., and H. O. Smith. 1975. Restriction endonucleases in the analysis and restructuring of DNA molecules. *Annual Review of Biochemistry* 44:273–93.

Nauta, H. J. W. 1979. A proposed conceptual reorganization of the basal ganglia and telencephalon. *Neuroscience* 4:1875–81.

Nauta, H. J. W. 1986. The relationship of the basal ganglia to the limbic system. In *Extrapyramidal Disorders*, edited by P. J. Vinken, G. W. Bruyn, and H. L. Klawans.

Pp. 19–31. Vol. 49 of *Handbook of Clinical Neurology*. New York: Elsevier Science Publishers.

Nauta, H. J. W., and M. Feirtag. 1986. *Fundamental Neuroanatomy*. New York: Freeman and Company.

Nauta, W. J. H., and V. B. Domesick. 1981. Ramifications of the limbic system. In *Psychiatry and Biology of the Human Brain*, edited by S. Matthysse. New York: Elsevier North Holland Biomedical Press.

Neel, J. V., and L. J. Schull. 1954. *Human Heredity*. Chicago: University of Chicago Press. Pp. 230–60.

Newcombe, R. G., D. A. Walker, and P. S. Harper. 1981. Factors influencing age at onset and duration of survival in Huntington's chorea. *Annals of Human Genetics* 45:387–96.

Norton, J. C. 1975. Patterns of neuropsychological test performance in Huntington's disease. *Journal of Nervous and Mental Disease* 161:276–79.

Nutt, J. G., and N. T. Morgan. 1983. Acute effects of scopolamine in Huntington's disease. *Advances in Neurology* 37:291–97.

Oepen, G., U. Mohr, K. Willmes, and U. Thoden. 1985. Huntington's disease: Visuomotor disturbance in patients and offspring. *Journal of Neurology, Neurosurgery, and Psychiatry* 48:426–33.

Oliver, J. E. 1970. Huntington's chorea in Northamptonshire. *British Journal of Psychiatry* 116:241–53.

Olney, J. W. 1969. Glutamate-induced retinal degeneration in neonatal mice. Electron-microscopy of acutely evolving lesion. *Journal of Neuropathology and Experimental Neurology* 28:455–74.

Omenn, G. S., J. G. Hall, and K. D. Hansen. 1980. Genetic counseling for adoptees at risk for specific inherited disorders. *American Journal of Medical Genetics* 5:157–64.

Oscar-Berman, M., D. S. Sax, and L. Opoliner. 1973. Effects of memory aids on hypothesis behavior and focusing in patients with Huntington's chorea. *Advances in Neurology* 1:717–28.

Osler, W. 1894. On chorea and choreiform affections. Philadelphia: Blackiston, Son and Company.

Osler, W. 1908. Historical note on hereditary chorea. In *Neurographs*. Vol. 1, 113–16. Edited by W. Browning. Brooklyn: Albert C. Huntington Publishing.

Ott, J. 1974. Estimation of the recombination fraction in human pedigrees: Efficient computation of the likelihood for human linkage studies. *American Journal of Human Genetics* 26:588–97.

Panse, F. 1942. Die Erbchorea: Eineklinisch-genetische Studie. Leipzig: Georg Thieme.

Pasik, P., T. Pasik, and M. DiFiglia. 1976. Quantitative aspects of neuronal organization in the neostriatum of the macaque monkey. In *The Basal Ganglia, Research Publications of the Association for Research in Nervous and Mental Disease*. Vol. 55, 57–90. Edited by M. D. Yahr. New York: Raven Press.

Pearlstein, L. S., C. B. Brill, and E. L. Mancall. 1982. Child abuse in Huntington's disease. *Pediatrics* 70:630–32.

Penney Jr., J. B., and A. B. Young. 1982. Quantitative autoradiography of neurotransmitter receptors in Huntington disease. *Neurology* (New York) 32:1391–95.

Penney Jr., J. B., and A. B. Young. 1986. Striatal inhomogeneities and basal ganglia function. *Movement Disorders* 1:3–15.

Penny, G. R., S. Afsharpour, and S. T. Kitai. 1986. The glutamate decarboxylase-, leucine enkephalin-, methionine enkephalin- and substance P-immunoreactive neurons in the neostriatum of the rat and cat: Evidence for partial population overlap. *Neuroscience* 17:1011–45.

Penny, G. R., H. T. Chang, and S. T. Kitai. 1986. Dual localization of [leu]-enkephalin and choline acetyltransferase in the rat basal ganglia. *Society for Neuroscience* 12:abstr. 362.10.

Pericak-Vance, M. A., P. M. Conneally, A. D. Merritt, R. P. Roos, J. M. Vance, P. L. Yu, I. A. Norton, Jr., and J. P. Artel. 1979. Genetic linkage in Huntington's disease. *Advances in Neurology* 23:59–72.

Pericak-Vance, M. A., R. C. Elston, P. M. Conneally, and D. V. Dawson. 1983. Age-of-onset heterogeneity in Huntington disease families. *American Journal of Medical Genetics* 14:49–59.

Perry, T. L., S. Hansen, D. Lesk, and M. Kloster. 1973. Amino acids in plasma, cerebrospinal fluid, and brain of patients with Huntington's chorea. *Advances in Neurology* 1:609–18.

Pincus, J. H., and A. Chutorian. 1967. Familial benign chorea with intention tremor: A clinical entity. *Journal of Pediatrics* 70:724–29.

Potegal, M. 1971. A note on spatial-motor deficits in patients with Huntington's disease: A test of a hypothesis. *Neuropsychologia* 9:233–35.

Quarrell, O. W. J., A. Tyler, G. Cole, and P. S. Harper. 1986. The problem of isolated cases of Huntington's disease in South Wales, 1974–1984. *Clinical Genetics* 30:331–37.

Ramig, L. A. 1986. Acoustic analyses of phonation in patients with Huntington's disease: Preliminary report. *Annals of Otology, Rhinology, and Laryngology* 95:288–93.

Reed, T. E., J. H. Chandler, E. M. Hughes, and R. T. Davidson. 1958. Huntington's chorea in Michigan: I. Demography and Genetics. *American Journal of Human Genetics* 10:201–25.

Reed, T. E., and J. V. Neel. 1959. Huntington's chorea in Michigan: II. Selection and mutation. *American Journal of Human Genetics* 11:107–36.

Reik, W., A. Collick, M. L. Norris, S. C. Barton, M. A. Surani. 1987. Genomic imprinting determines methylation of parental alleles in transgenic mice. *Nature* 328:248–51.

Reisine, T. D., J. Z. Fields, L. Z. Stern, P. C. Johnson, E. D. Bird, H. I. Yamamura. 1977. Alterations in dopaminergic receptors in Huntington's disease. *Life Sciences* 21:1123–28.

Richfield, E. K., R. Twyman, and S. Berent. 1987. Neurological syndrome following bilateral damage to the head of the caudate nuclei. *Annals of Neurology* 22:768–71.

Robins, L. N., J. E. Helzer, M. M. Weissman, H. Orvaschel, E. Gruenberg, J. D. Burke, and D. A. Regier. 1984. Lifetime prevalence of specific psychiatric disorders in three sites. *Archives of General Psychiatry* 41:949–58.

Robinson, M. B., and J. T. Coyle. 1987. Glutamate and related acidic excitatory neurotransmitters: From basic science to clinical application. *Federation of Societies for Experimental Biology* 1:446–55.

Roos, R. A. C. 1986. Neuropathology of Huntington's chorea. In *Extrapyramidal Disorders,* edited by P. J. Vinken, G. W. Bruyn, and H. L. Klawans. Pp. 315–26. Vol. 49 of *Handbook of Clinical Neurology.* New York: Elsevier Science Publishers.

Roos, R. A. C., G. T. A. Bots, and J. Hermans. 1985. Neuronal nuclear membrane indentation and astrocyte/neuron ratio in Huntington's disease: A quantitative electron microscope study. *Journal fuer Hirnforschung* 26:689–93.

Roos, R. A. C., J. F. M. Pruyt, J. de Vries, and G. T. A. Bots. 1985. Neuronal distribution in the putamen in Huntington's disease. *Journal of Neurology, Neurosurgery, and Psychiatry* 48:422–25.

Rosenberg, R. N. 1980. A science and practice of clinical medicine. In *Neurology.* Vol. 5. Edited by J. M. Diepschy, and R. N. Rosenberg. New York: Grune and Stratton.

Salazar, A. M., J. Grafman, S. Schlesselman, S. C. Vance, J. P. Mohr, M. Carpenter, P. Pevsner, C. Ludlow, and H. Weingartner. 1986. Penetrating war injuries of the basal forebrain: Neurology and cognition. *Neurology* 36:459–65.

Sanberg, P. R., and J. T. Coyle. 1984. Scientific approaches to Huntington's disease. *Critical Reviews in Clinical Neurobiology* 1:1–44.

Sandell, J. H., A. M. Graybiel, and M. F. Chesselet. 1986. A new enzyme marker for striatal compartmentalization: NADPH diaphorase activity in the caudate nucleus and putamen of the cat. *Journal of Comparative Neurology* 243:326–34.

Sapienza, C., A. C. Paterson, J. Rossant, R. Balling. 1987. Degree of methylation of transgenes is dependent on gamete of origin. *Nature* 328:251–54.

Saugstad, L., and O. Odegard. 1986. Huntington's chorea in Norway. *Psychological Medicine* 16:39–48.

Sax, D. S., B. O'Donnell, N. Butters, L. Menzer, K. Montgomery, and H. L. Kayne. 1983. Computer tomographic, neurologic, and neuropsychological correlates of Huntington's disease. *International Journal of Neuroscience* 18:21–36.

Schott, G. D. 1986. Induction of involuntary movements by peripheral trauma: An analogy with causalgia. *Lancet* (September 27), 712–16.

Schwarcz, R., and C. Kohler. 1983. Differential vulnerability of central neurons of the rat to quinolinic acid. *Neuroscience Letters* 38:85–90.

Schwarcz, R., C. Kohler, R. M. Mangano, and A. N. Neophytides. 1981. Glutamate-induced neuronal degeneration: Studies on the role of glutamate re-uptake. *Advances in Biochemical Psychopharmacology* 27:403–12.

Scrimgeour, E. M. 1980. Huntington's disease in two New Britain families. *Journal of Medical Genetics* 17:197–202.

Shaw, M., and A. Caro. 1982. The mutation rate to Huntington's chorea. *Journal of Medical Genetics* 19:161–67.

Shokeir, M. H. K. 1975a. Investigations on Huntington's disease in the Canadian prairies: I. Prevalence. *Clinical Genetics* 7:345–48.

Shokeir, M. H. K. 1975b. Investigation on Huntington's disease in the Canadian prairies: II. Fecundity and fitness. *Clinical Genetics* 7:349–53.

Shoulson, I., and S. Fahn. 1979. Huntington's disease: Clinical care and evaluation. *Neurology* 29:1–3.

Shoulson, I., D. Goldblatt, M. Charlton, and R. J. Joynt. 1978. Huntington's disease: Treatment with muscimal, a GABA-mimetic drug. *Annals of Neurology* 4:279–84.

Shoulson, I., R. Kurlan, A. Rubin, D. Glodblatt, J. Behr, C. Miller, J. Kennedy, K. Bamford, E. Caine, D. Kido, S. Plumb, C. Odoroff. 1989. Assessment of functional capacity in neuro-degenerative movement disorders: Huntington's disease as a prototype. In *Quantification of Neurological Deficits*, edited by T. Munsat. Stoneham: Butterworth Publishers.

Simmons, J. T., B. Pastakia, T. N. Chase, and C. W. Shults. 1986. Magnetic resonance imaging in Huntington disease. *American Journal of Neuroradiology* 7:25–28.

Sjogren, T. 1936. Verer bungsmedizinische untersuchungen uber Huntingtonsche chorea in einer Schwedischen bauernpopulation. *Zeitschriftfuer Menschliche Vererbungs- und Konstitutions Lehre* 19:132–65.

Smith, B. A., J. McMahon, J. J. Wasmuth. 1988. Isolation of three cDNA clones from a small region of 4p16.3 known to contain the Huntington's disease gene. *American Journal of Human Genetics* 43:abstract 803.

Starkstein, S., E. J. Boston, and R. G. Robinson. 1988. Mechanisms of mania following brain injury: Twelve case reports and review of the literature. *Journal of Nervous and Mental Disease* 176:87–100.

Starkstein, S. E., J. Brandt, S. Folstein, M. Strauss, M. L. Berthier, G. D. Pearlson, D. Wong, A. McDonnell, and M. Folstein. 1988. Neuropsychologic and neuropathologic correlates in Huntington's disease. *Journal of Neurology, Neurosurgery, and Psychiatry* 51:1259–63.

Starkstein, S. E., J. Brandt, S. Folstein, M. Strauss, A. McDonnell, and M. Folstein. 1988. Brain atrophy in Huntington's disease: Correlations with clinical and neuropsychological findings. *Neuroradiology* 359, abstract 4.

Starkstein, S. E., S. E. Folstein, J. Brandt, A. McDonnell, and M. Folstein. Brain atrophy in Huntington's disease: A CT-scan study. *Neuroradiology*. In press.

Starkstein, S. E., R. G. Robinson, M. L. Berthier, R. M. Parikh, and T. R. Price. 1988. Differential mood changes following basal ganglia vs thalamic lesions. *Archives of Neurology* 45:725–30.

Starkstein, S. E., R. G. Robinson, and T. R. Price. 1987. Comparison of cortical and subcortical lesions in the production of poststroke mood disorders. *Brain* 110:1045–59.

Starr, A. 1967. A disorder of rapid eye movements in Huntington's chorea. *Brain* 90:545–64.

Stevens, D., and M. Parsonage. 1969. Mutation in Huntington's chorea. *Journal of Neurology, Neurosurgery, and Psychiatry* 32:140–43.

Stewart, J. T., M. L. Mounts, and R. L. Clark, Jr. 1987. Aggressive behavior in Huntington's disease: Treatment with propranolol. *Journal of Clinical Psychiatry* 48:106–8.

Still, C. N. 1977. Huntington's chorea in South Carolina: Natural history and clinical features. *Neurologica, Neurocirurgia, Psiquiatria* 18(2–3 suppl.):193–98.

Stone, T. T., and E. I. Falstein. 1938. Pathology of Huntington's chorea, II. *Journal of Nervous and Mental Disease* 88:602–26.

Strauss, M. E., and J. Brandt. 1986. Attempt at preclinical identification of Huntington's disease using the WAIS. *Journal of Clinical and Experimental Neuropsychology* 8:210–18.

Stuss, D., and D. F. Benson, eds. 1986. *The Frontal Lobes*. New York: Raven Press.

Suchowersky, O., M. Hayden, W. R. W. Martin, D. K. Li, M. Bergstrom, R. Marrop, J. Rogers, C. Sayre, and B. D. Pate. 1984. Benign heredity chorea: Clinical, radiological and PET findings. *Canadian Journal of the Neurological Sciences* 11:329.

Taylor, A. E., J. A. Saint-Cyr, and A. E. Lang. 1986. Frontal lobe dysfunction in Parkinson's disease. *Brain* 109:845–83.

Tellez-Nagel, I., A. B. Johnson, and R. D. Terry. 1973. Ultrastructural and histochemical study of cerebral biopsies in Huntington's chorea. *Advances in Neurology* 1:387–98.

Thompson, W. D., H. Orvaschel, B. A. Prusoff, and K. K. Kidd. 1982. An evaluation of the family history method for ascertaining psychiatric disorders. *Archives of General Psychiatry* 39:53–58.

Trautner, R. J., J. L. Cummings, S. L. Read, and D. F. Benson. 1988. Idiopathic basal ganglia calcification and organic mood disorder. *American Journal of Psychiatry* 145:350–53.

Tulipan, N., S. Huang, W. O. Whetsell, and G. S. Allen. 1986. Neonatal striatal grafts prevent lethal syndrome produced by bilateral intrastriatal injection of kainic acid. *Brain Research* 377:163–67.

Tyler, A., and P. S. Harper. 1983. Attitudes of subjects at risk and their relatives towards genetic counselling in Huntington's chorea. *Journal of Medical Genetics* 20:179–88.

Tyler, A., P. S. Harper, K. Davies, and R. G. Newcombe. 1983. Family break-down and stress in Huntington's chorea. *Journal of Biosocial Science* 15:127–38.

Tyler, A., P. S. Harper, D. A. Walker, K. Davies, and R. G. Newcombe. 1982. The socioeconomic burden of Huntington's chorea in South Wales. *Journal of Biosocial Science* 14:379–89.

U.S. Department of Health and Human Services. 1986. *Disability Evaluation under Social Security*. No. 05-10089. Social Security Administration.

U.S. Department of Health, Education, and Welfare. 1977. Huntington's Disease and Its Consequences. Report: Commission for the Control of (1977): Vol. I–IV.: Technical Report.

Vonsattel, J. P., R. H. Meyers, T. J. Stevens, R. J. Ferrante, E. D. Bird, E. P. Richardson, Jr. 1985. Neuropathological classification of Huntington's disease. *Journal of Neuropathology and Experimental Neurology* 44:559–77.

Walker, D. A., P. S. Harper, C. E. C. Wells, A. Tyler, K. Davies, and R. G. Newcombe. 1981. Huntington's chorea in South Wales: A genetic and epidemiological study. *Clinical Genetics* 19:213–21.

Walker, F. O., A. B. Young, J. B. Penney, K. Dovorini-Zis, and I. Shoulson. 1984. Benzodiazepine and GABA receptors in early Huntington's disease. *Neurology* (Cleveland) 34:1237–40.

Wallace, D. C. 1972. Huntington's chorea in Queensland: A not uncommon disease. *Medical Journal of Australia* 1:299–307.

Wallace, D. C. 1987. Maternal genes: Mitochondrial diseases. In *Medical and Experimental Genetics: A Perspective*. Vol. 23, no. 3, 137–90. Edited by V. A. McKusick, T. H. Roderick, J. Mori, and N. W. Paul. March of Dimes Birth Defects Foundation. New York: Alan R. Liss, Inc.

Wallace, D. C., and A. C. Hall. 1972. Evidence of genetic heterogeneity in Huntington's chorea. *Journal of Neurology, Neurosurgery, and Psychiatry* 35:789–800.

Walshe, T. M., and C. Leonard. 1985. Persistent vegetative state: Extension of the syndrome to include chronic disorders. *Archives of Neurology* 42:1045–47.

Wasmuth, J. J., J. Hewitt, B. Smith, D. Allard, J. L. Haines, D. Skarecky, E. Partlow, and M. R. Hayden. 1988. A highly polymorphic locus very tightly linked to the Huntington's disease gene. *Nature* 332:734–36.

Weingartner, H., E. D. Caine, and M. H. Ebert. 1979. Imagery, encoding, and retrieval of information from memory: Some specific encoding-retrieval changes in Huntington's disease. *Journal of Abnormal Psychology* 88:52–58.

Wendt, G. G., and D. Drohm. 1972. *Die Huntingtonsche Chorea: Eine Populationsgenetische Studie. Fortschritte der allgemeinen und klinischen Humangenetik.* Band IV. Herausgegeben von P. E. Becker, W. Lenz, F. Vogel, ans G. G. Wendt. Stuttgart: Georg Thieme Verlag.

Went, L. N., M. Vegter-Van der Vlis, G. W. Bruyn, and W. S. Volkers. 1983. Huntington's chorea in the Netherlands: The problem of genetic heterogeneity. *Annals of Human Genetics* 47:205–14.

Went, L. N., M. Vegter-Van der Vlis, W. Volkers, and H. Collewijn. 1975. Huntington's chorea. In *Early Diagnosis and Prevention of Genetic Diseases.* Edited by L. N. Went, C. Vermeij-Keers, and A. G. J. M. Van der Linden. Leiden: Leiden University Press.

Wexler, N. 1975. Living out the dying (The counselor and genetic disease: Huntington's disease as a model). ERIC reports, National Institute of Education, DHEW.

Wexler, N. S. 1979. Perceptual-motor, cognitive, and emotional characteristics of persons at risk for Huntington's disease. *Advances in Neurology* 23:257–71.

Wheeler, J. S., D. S. Sax, R. J. Krane, and M. B. Siroky. 1985. Vesico-urethral function in Huntington's chorea. *British Journal of Urology* 57:63–66.

Whitehouse, P. J., B. E. Jones, R. R. Trifiletti, S. E. Folstein, D. L. Price, and M. J. Kuhar. 1985. Neurotransmitter receptor alterations in Huntington's disease: Autoradiographic studies. *Annals of Neurology* 18:202–10.

Whittier, J. R. 1947. Ballism and the subthalamic nucleus (nucleus hypothalamicus; corpus Luysi). *Archives of Neurology and Psychiatry* 58:672–92.

Wilson, R. S., and D. C. Garron. 1979. Cognitive and affective aspects of Huntington's disease. *Advances in Neurology* 23:193–201.

Wittes, J. T., T. Colton, and V. W. Sidel. 1974. Capture-recapture methods for assessing the completeness of case ascertainment when using multiple information sources. *Journal of Chronic Diseases* 27:25–36.

Wright, H. H., C. N. Still, and R. K. Abramson. 1981. Huntington's disease in black kindreds in South Carolina. *Archives of Neurology* 38:412–14.

Young, A. B., H. S. Pan, B. J. Ciliax, and J. B. Penney. 1984. GABA and benzodiazepine receptors in basal ganglia function. *Neuroscience Letters* 47:361–67.

Young, A. B., J. B. Penney, M. Z. Hollingsworth, J. Teener, J. Stern, J. Gusella, P. St. George-Hyslop, W. Hobbs, J. Rothley, and A. Betley. 1988. Genetic linkage analysis, glucose metabolism and neurologic examination: Comparison in persons at risk for Huntington's disease (HD). *Neurology* 359, abstract 2.

Young, A. B., J. T. Greenamyre, Z. Hollingsworth, R. Albin, C. D'Amato, I. Shoulson, and J. B. Penney. 1988. MNDA receptor losses in putamen from patients with Huntington's disease. *Science* 241:981–83.

Young, A. B., J. B. Penney, S. Starosta-Rubinstein, D. Markel, S. Berent, J. Rothley, A. Betley, and R. Hichwa. 1987. Normal caudate glucose metabolism in persons at risk for Huntington's disease. *Archives of Neurology* 44:254–57.

Young, A. B., I. Shoulson, J. B. Penney, S. Starosta-Rubinstein, F. Gomez, H.

Travers, M. A. Ramos-Arroyo, S. R. Snodgrass, E. Bonilla, H. Moreno, and N. S. Wexler. 1986. Huntington's disease in Venezuela: Neurologic features and functional decline. *Neurology* 36:244–49.

Youngman, S., M. Sarfarazi, O. W. J. Quarrell, P. M. Conneally, K. Gibbons, P. S. Harper, D. J. Shaw, R. E. Tanzi, M. R. Wallace, and J. F. Gusella. 1986. Studies of a DNA marker (G8) genetically linked to Huntington disease in British families. *Human Genetics* 73:333–39.

Youngman, S., D. J. Shaw, M. Bucan, M. Zimmer, M. MacDonald, C. Gilliam, B. Smith, J. Wasmuth, J. Gusella, A. Frischauf, H. Learch, P. S. Harper. 1988. D4S90 (D5), a DNA segment in close proximity to Huntington's disease, is the most terminally located probe on the short arm of chromosome 4. *American Journal of Human Genetics* 43:abstract 651.

Yung, C. Y. 1984. A review of clinical trials of lithium in neurology. *Pharmacology Biochemistry and Behavior* 21(suppl. 1):57–64.

Zweig, R. M., S. J. Koven, J. C. Hedreen, N. E. Maestri, H. H. Kazazian, and S. E. Folstein. Linkage to the HD locus in a family with unusual clinical and pathological features. *Annals of Neurology*, in press.

Index

Acetylcholine
  aspiny interneurons, 75
  in HD, 81
  in striosomes, 75
Activities of daily living, documentation of,
  199–201
Adoption
  informing adoptive parents, 131–32
  obtaining family history, 131–32
Advanced disease
  cognitive capacity in, 35
  communication in, 28
  diagnosis in, 139
  feeding in, 28
  motor disorder in, 27–28
  as a persistent vegetative state, 28
  signs in, 138–39
Affective disorder, 54–56
  age at onset, relation to, 55, 112
  case example, 50–51
  confusion with schizophrenia, 49
  delusions in, 54
  diagnostic criteria, 54
  familial aggregation of, 61–62, 112
  major vs. "reactive" depression, 54, 55–56
  neuropathologic hypotheses, 63–64
  in persons at risk, 173–74
  pharmacologic management, 163–64
  as a presenting feature, 51, 55
  prevalence, 61–63
  racial variation in, 61–62
Africans. See Blacks
Aggression. See Irritability
Alcoholism, 59
Anxiety, 58, 163, 173–74
Apathy, 34–35, 52

Ascertainment of cases
  incomplete, 90, 91–92
  prevalence influenced by methods for, 91
  sources of, 92–93, 102–4
Aspiny neurons, 68
  in HD, 80–81
  neurochemistry of, 75
Ataxia. See Gait
At-risk for HD, characteristics of persons,
  170–75
  antisocial behavior, 173–74
  cognition, 174
  concerns about employment, 155, 172
  neurologic features, 174–75
  personality features, 170–71
  preparation for illness, 155
  psychiatric disorder 173, 177
  psychologic burdens, 158–59, 171–72
At risk for HD, care of persons, 152–53,
  175–78. See also Genetic Testing
  disclosing risk, 131–32, 152–53, 175–76
  genetic counseling, 177–78, 213–14
  psychotherapy, 177
  prevalence of persons, 98–99

Basal ganglia. See also Striatum
  definition, 68, 73
  functions of, 67
Benzodiazepine receptors. See Gamma-
  aminobutyric Acid
Blacks
  age at onset, 112, 137
  case finding, 102–3
  clinical features in, 136–37
  prevalence, 95–97
Brain banks, 10, 212

Case examples
  cognitive disorder, 32–33
  diagnosis, 125–27
  emotional disorder, 50–51
  epidemiology, 89–90
  genetics, 107–8
  movement disorder, 13–16
  neuropathology, 76–77
  presymptomatic testing, 169–70
  treatment, 150–51
Caudate nucleus. *See* Striatum
Center Without Walls for HD, 9–10
Child abuse, 59, 159
Chorea
  in advanced disease, 27–28
  ballismus, as distinguished from, 75
  definition of, 17
  dopamine system, relationship to, 30–31, 84
  as a presenting sign, 16–17, 132–33
  response to neuroleptics, 160–61
  during sleep, 20
  severity of, relative to duration, 17–19
  subthalamic nucleus, relationship to, 30–31
  in Sydenham's chorea, 19
  in tardive dyskinesia, 29–30
  variation with setting, 19, 133
Clinical features, 2–6, 13–64, 132–40. *See also* Case examples
  age at death, 4
  age at onset, 4–5
  causes of death, 6
  duration of illness, 5
  Huntington's description of, 1–4
  natural history, 138–40
  triad of, 2, 13–64
Clinical features, standardized documentation of, 189–201
  activities of daily living, 199–201
  Mini-Mental Status Examination (MMSE), 196–97
  neurological examination, 189–95
  onset of signs and symptoms, 197–99
Clinical-pathological correlations, 83–84
  with cognitive disorder, 46–67, 83–84
  with emotional disorder, 63–64, 84
  with motor disorder, 30–31, 83–84
Cognitive impairment. *See also* Mini-Mental Status Examination (MMSE)
  assessment in the clinic, 35–40
  attention and concentration, 45

  case example, 32–33
  neuropathologic hypotheses, 46–47
  presentation at home and work, 33–34, 134–35
  relationship to duration of illness, 33–37
  relationship to education, 36, 37
  relationship to motor disorder, 29
  set changing, 34, 46
  subcortical dementia, 32, 35
  variability in, 36–37, 134–35
  visuospatial impairment, 44, 45–46
Community surveys. *See* Prevalence
Congressional Commission on HD, 9–10
Conneally, Michael, national HD roster, 10, 120
Corpus striatum. *See* Striatum
Cortical-subcortical circuits, 70–73, 76, 83–84

Death, age at, 4
Delusions. *See* Affective disorder; Schizophrenia
Depression. *See* Affective disorder
Diagnosis, 125–48
Differential diagnosis. *See* Chapters 2, 3, and 4
Disclosure
  acceptance of, 151–52
  of advanced disease, 139
  of blacks, 136–37
  case example, 125–27
  course of illness, 138–40
  of juvenile onset HD, 135–36
  of late onset HD, 137
  mis-, 141–43
  with a negative family history, 109, 127, 129, 143–44
  of PET in, 144–47
  use of CT, MRI in, 143, 144–46
  use of genetic linkage to confirm, 184–85
  use of neuropathology in, 147
  use of paternity testing in, 143–44
  variations in presentation, 132–35
Diagnostic criteria, 125–48
  influence on prevalence estimates, 101–2
  for psychiatric disorders in HD, 53–54, 202–7
Differential diagnosis, 140–43
  Alzheimer's disease, 35, 37–40, 45
  Parkinson's disease, 21
  senile chorea, 137

in feeding, 25–26, 161–62
in gait, 26, 155, 157
motor latency and impersistence, 21
predominance in advanced illness, 27–28
as a presenting sign, 133–34
relation to duration of illness, 26
in speech, 24–25, 162
Voluntary organizations
addresses, 211–12
family support by, 158
Hereditary Disease Foundation, 9
Huntington's Disease Society of America, 212
origins, 8–9
use in community surveys, 103

WAIS. *See* Intelligence tests
Westphal variant
as example of distinction between voluntary and involuntary movements, 28
definition of, 17
dystonia in, 20
fine motor coordination in, 23
tremor and myoclonus in, 20
Wexler, Milton, 9
Wexler, Nancy
director of Congressional Commission, 9
Venezuela Project, 10, 95, 120
Wills Foundation, 8. *See also* Congressional Commission